THE SUGAR ADDICT'S TOTAL RECOVERY PROGRAM

By Kathleen DesMaisons, Ph.D.

Potatoes Not Prozac
The Sugar Addict's Total Recovery Program

THE SUGAR ADDICT'S

Total

RECOVERY PROGRAM

Kathleen DesMaisons, Ph.D.

THE BALLANTINE PUBLISHING GROUP

NEW YORK

The recommendations in this book are not intended to replace or conflict with advice given to you by your physician or other health care professional. If you have a preexisting medical or psychological condition, or are currently taking medication, consult with your physician before adopting the suggestions in this book. Following these dietary suggestions may impact certain types of medications. Any change in your dosage should be made only in cooperation with your prescribing physician.

A Ballantine Book
Published by The Ballantine Publishing Group
Copyright © 2000 by Kathleen DesMaisons, Ph.D.

www.randomhouse.com/BB/

LIBRARY OF CONGRESS CATALOGING-IN-PUBLICATION DATA
DesMaisons, Kathleen.
The sugar addict's total recovery program / Kathleen DesMaisons.—1st ed.
p.   cm.
Includes bibliographical references and index.
ISBN 0-345-44132-X
1. Sugar-free diet.   2. Compulsive eating—Diet therapy.
3. Depression, Mental—Diet therapy.   I. Title.
RM237.85.D473 2000
613.2'5—dc21   00-059907

Manufactured in the United States of America

First Edition: December 2000

10 9 8 7 6 5 4 3 2 1

Mother, thank you for your continuing love. Your guidance makes it work.

Contents

Introduction   3

1. Why You Are Different   13
Criteria for Addiction • Sugar Sensitivity: The Three
Components • Carbohydrate Sensitivity • Brain
Chemicals • Sex Differences in Brain Chemicals • The
Three-Legged Stool • Why Other Eating Plans Haven't
Worked for Sugar Addicts

2. The Solution   41
Introducing the Seven Steps • Why the Steps Are in This
Order • Getting Ready to Start • Sugar Feelings • Keeping
Things Simple • The Best Way to Use This Recovery
Program

3. Getting Started: Steps 1 and 2   55
Step 1. Eat Breakfast with Protein Every Day • Ten Breakfast
Ideas • Fast Food Breakfast Choices • A Shopping List to
Cope with Chaos • Step 2. Journal What You Eat and How
You Feel • Learning to Read Your Body

4. **Getting Steady: Steps 3 and 4** 70

Step 3. Eat Three Meals a Day with Protein • Regular Protein Is Crucial • What Is a Meal? • Have Sweets with Your Meal and Don't Worry About It • Why Only Three Meals? And Why No Snacks? • Grocery Shopping • Step 4. Eat a Potato Before Bed • Take Three Vitamins

5. **Getting the Details Sorted Out: Answers to Your Questions** 90

Is This a High-Fat Diet? • Isn't This Too Much Protein? • Questions on How Eating the Potato Works • Questions on Choosing and Preparing Your Potato • Questions on the Timing of Your Potato • Questions on How to Make the Plan Work

6. **Creating a Routine** 107

Doing Regular Life • What to Do If You Slip • No More Fighting—Mastery • Planning Your Food: What's Your Style? • A Little Exercise Always Helps • Water, Water All the Time • Why Some Stuff Will Help • Trying New Foods—Starting to Explore • Planning for Downtimes

7. **Halfway There: Step 5** 131

Step 5. Shift from White Foods to Brown Foods • Don't Forget the Potato! • What to Eat in This Phase • Finding New Comfort Foods

8. **Taking the Sugars Out: Step 6** 150

Setting the Stage • Having Second Thoughts • Planning for the Big Day • Being Attentive to Your Plan • The Sugar/ Alcohol Dilemma • Final Preparations • What to Eat • Life After Detox

9. **Staying with the Program over Time: Step 7** 176

Socializing Without Sugars • How Your Ambivalence Can Affect Your No • Staying Out of Trouble • Getting Support • What to Do When You're Cranky • What About Relapse? • Creating Other Kinds of Comfort

10. **Special Situations**   **196**
    Making Contingency Plans • Going Out to Eat • Further
    Plans for Special Occasions • Traveling • Other Special
    Situations • In Closing

11. **Recipes from Fellow Travelers**   **216**
    Breakfast • Lunch • Dinner • Breads • Soups and Side
    Dishes • Salad Dressings • Treats and Desserts

    Bibliography   **253**

    Resources   **263**

    Acknowledgments   **267**

    Index   **269**

THE SUGAR
ADDICT'S
TOTAL
RECOVERY
PROGRAM

Introduction

Are you a sugar addict? Have you ever wondered why you love sweet foods so much? Does chocolate run your life more than you want to admit? Do you joke about being a "sweet freak"? Does it ever scare you to feel so compulsive about wanting sugar? The questions listed below will help you understand what it means to be a sugar addict. When I say "sweet foods," I mean coffee or tea with sugar, cookies, cakes, candy, cereal, soda, ice cream, sweet rolls, energy bars, lattes iced with syrups, chocolate, or any food that you know is sweetened with sugar, honey, or artificial sweeteners.

❏ **Have you ever tried to cut down or control your use of sweet foods?**
Have you ever picked a certain day and said, "Starting Monday I am not going to have chocolate"?

Have you ever been secretly delighted when you are out to dinner and your friends order dessert and urge you to join them?

❑ **Are you using more sweet foods than ever before?**

Have you ever realized that you used to get one Butterfinger candy bar, but now you buy three at a time?

Do you find yourself stopping at the convenience store for bread and milk *and* M&M's?

❑ **If you don't have your regular "dose" of sugar, do you get irritable and cranky?**

Have you ever been in a meeting at work and found yourself unable to pay attention to the agenda because you are thinking about your afternoon double latte?

Have you ever been frantic when you arrive at your friends' house for the weekend to discover they have *no* sweets in the house and you have no car?

❑ **Have you ever gotten upset when someone ate your special food?**

Have you ever felt silent rage and panic when you have gone to the refrigerator for the last of the cream pie and discovered someone had eaten it?

Have you ever kept a stash of chocolate in your underwear drawer and been horrified when your daughter found it?

Are you unable to keep a stash anywhere because you eat it first?

❑ **Have you ever lied about how much sweet food you eat?**

Have you ever told your kids you don't know where the last box of Girl Scout Thin Mints is when you know you ate them and put the box in the bottom of the trash?

Have you ever said, "I don't know what happened to it" when you know perfectly well you ate it?

❑ **Have you ever gone out of your way to get something sweet?**

Have you ever gone far out of your way to stop at the coffee shop for your favorite drink and sweet roll?

Have you ever chosen a restaurant based on the quality of its desserts even though it's an hour's drive away?

❏ **Have you ever binged on sweet or white flour foods?**

Have you ever told yourself you were going to have just a bite of ice cream and ended up eating the whole quart all by yourself?

Have you ever gotten a special cake for the potluck on the weekend and ended up eating the whole thing yourself?

❏ **Have you ever felt you had a sugar hangover?**

Have you ever crawled through the morning with a headache and crankiness that is immediately relieved when you have something sweet?

❏ **Is it impossible to "just say no" to sweet foods?**

Do you feel inordinately relieved when you finally get your sweets?

Have you ever made a cover noise like coughing, singing, or humming while you opened the cabinet door to get your sweets?

❏ **Is sugar controlling your life?**

Are you ashamed and fearful that you will always be out of control? Would you be horrified to have your friends know how you answered any of these questions?

If you answered yes to two or more of the questions in bold-face, you are probably a sugar addict. You are reading the right book. If you answered yes to all the questions, you have come home to the right place! While you may not let yourself admit openly to these secrets, you know they are true. You know that you have hidden candy wrappers under the trash so no one would know you had eaten another. You know you have sneaked cookies before the family came home so they wouldn't know who ate the last ones. You know you have lied, cheated, and stolen for your "drug" of choice. These are signs of addiction, but until now you may not have let yourself think about applying these words to your relationship to sugar.

I understand how powerful these feelings are. I would have answered yes to every question in my sugar days. I am a sugar addict like you, but now I am in recovery from my sugar addiction. This recovery has saved my life, and I want to share with you the solutions I have found. I have deep compassion for what you are dealing with and want to bring you the healing and radiance that my recovery has given me.

My father was an alcoholic and died of alcoholism when I was only sixteen. I grew up with all the classic symptoms of being the child of an alcoholic. I had to stop drinking in my early twenties, but I still had a powerful interest in sweet things. I needed them. I planned my life around them. I kept a supply, got upset if someone ate my goods, and knew the best places to get my "drugs." Even though until recently other people discounted the idea of a sugar addiction similar to an addiction to alcohol or drugs, I knew better. I knew my addiction to sweets was running my life.

At first, though, I thought the primary problem was my weight. I sincerely believed that if I just lost weight, everything would be okay. But over time, I came to see that the story of my weight was far bigger than just too many pounds—it was part of the story of my sugar addiction. I didn't realize it, but my sugar addiction was associated with my mood swings, depression, fatigue, fuzzy thinking, PMS, impulsivity, and unpredictable temper. I had no idea that all these things could be connected to what I was eating. After all, I was just eating sugar, not using heroin or alcohol.

I finally came to understand my own addiction through my professional work with addicts and alcoholics. I moved to California in the mid-eighties after an active career in public health, looking for a way to continue my long-standing commitment to helping others. Eventually I started and became director of an alcohol and drug treatment center, not then understanding how that would shape my own need for recovery.

Unaware that addiction treatment historically had at best a 25 percent success rate, I almost immediately became concerned about the lack of success we were having in our treatments. Six months after we began the center, I started looking for variables that might improve treatment outcomes. Initially, I looked at the issues that have traditionally been thought of as important in treatment: length of time in treatment; skill of the counselor; group versus individual work; twelve-step program involvement. None of them seemed to have any particular impact on our clients' ability to stay clean and sober.

During this time, I had changed my own eating because I wanted to lose weight. I had started on a diet that was very similar to what you will be reading about in this book: no sugar, moderate amounts of complex carbs, more protein, and regular meals. The results stunned me. Not only did I lose weight, I felt incredible. My cravings went away. My mood swings disappeared. I felt focused and clear and excited about life. I stopped feeling compulsive about food and sweets. These changes convinced me that something more than weight loss was going on. I had dieted before but had never felt like this. *This* felt like recovery. As a result, I got really interested in the relationship between diet and addiction.

I started to ask my clients about their diets as well as their patterns of drinking and using. While my clients were drinking or using, few of them cared about sweets. As soon as they got sober, however, their interest in sweets and refined carbohydrates like bread and pasta skyrocketed. The more they had, the more they wanted. Although many were sober, they still acted addictively toward their sweets. Their behavior resembled their old drinking patterns. They continued to be moody, impulsive, and irritable even though they had stopped drinking. Historically, these behaviors have been attributed to detoxification from alcohol or a state called a dry drunk. Because of my own experience with diet and mood, however, I suspected they stemmed from something biochemical. My clients were eating in the same way I had been eating. We had the same moods and emotional symptoms. Maybe, I thought, we shared a similar brain chemistry. Maybe we all were sugar addicts.

During this same time, seemingly by chance, I came across an article in an obscure journal that made a connection between alcoholism and sugar. The article suggested that there could be a correlation between diet and the ability to achieve sobriety. Because of my own personal history and what I was seeing with my clients, I intuitively felt that this connection had to be true and thought it might even be the link I sought for improving treatment outcomes in our clinic.

I followed my intuition. Drawing on my own experience, I developed a food plan for my clinic clients. When they followed the food plan, the number of people getting and staying clean and sober increased dramatically. During this same period I also maintained a private practice helping people make life changes. While the clients at the clinic were predominantly alcoholic men, my private clients were mostly overweight women who were depressed, dealing with mood swings, chaos in their lives, and low self-esteem. I started to ask them, too, about what they ate, which surprised them. After all, they were there to talk about what they felt, not about what they ate. I was floored to discover that their diets were very similar to the way I had been eating before I changed my diet. They skipped meals, ate huge amounts of carbohydrates, and basically lived on sugar. But they were willing to try almost anything to get better, even if they had to change what they ate and when they ate it.

As my private clients began to use the same food plan I had developed for the clinic, they experienced the same miraculous turnaround my clinic clients and I had: their depression lifted; they got clear, focused, and purposeful; and many lost weight. All were excited by the changes they experienced with what we called "doing the food."

I was so impressed by what I saw happening with my clients that I wanted to understand better why this plan was working so well. I decided to go back to school for a Ph.D. I gave up my full-time job, sold my house, and moved into a one-room apartment. I wasn't at all perturbed by the fact that I was fifty years old and committing to a whole new career path. I knew I was onto something and I was willing to put my money where my mouth was.

I put together a doctoral committee of experts in the fields of nutrition, public health, alcoholism, and neurochemistry, and together, we mapped out what I needed to learn.

As I read more and more scientific literature, I learned that sugar evokes a brain chemical called beta-endorphin—the very same chemical evoked by alcohol or heroin. Sugar could in fact cause the same chemical and mood effects in the body, albeit on a less intense level, as some of the most addictive substances in the world!

At the time I was doing my research, the scientific connection between sugar and addiction couldn't be found all in one place under "sugar addiction." There were bits and pieces and clues in the literature about alcoholism, heroin, depression, eating disorders, and nutrition. So I collected pieces of the puzzle from each field. I started reading information on the treatment of heroin addiction with a different eye. Heroin is one of a class of drugs called opioids that affect the beta-endorphin system within the brain. Substituting the word "sugar" for "opioids" led to some powerful insights. I read this line in my substance abuse text: "post-addict volunteers usually experience an elevation of mood and an increased sense of self-esteem" when they take opioids.

The idea that opioids and opioid-like substances such as sugar could affect self-esteem had an electrifying effect on me. I remember reading that line and feeling the hair on the back of my neck stand up. If sugar created an opioid effect, it would enhance self-esteem. No wonder my clients and I were drawn to it! I felt as if I was building a case for a theory of sugar addiction. Sugar addiction could be a real, physiological state and changing the diet could be a way to treat it.

I also wanted to know why sugar addiction developed in certain people. I developed a theory that a condition I called sugar sensitivity could explain why certain people were more vulnerable to the effects of alcohol and drugs than others. My doctoral study focused on the relationship between sugar sensitivity and alcoholism. Eventually, I expanded the theory to include sugar addiction as a symptom of sugar sensitivity. My doctoral work and my clinical practice demonstrate that diet can be an effective treatment for alcoholism and drug addiction as well as sugar addiction. Incorporating this food plan into our treatment program had had a huge impact on the success of the program: 90 percent of the alcoholic clients who used the food protocol graduated from the treatment program, and 92 percent of the graduates were still clean and sober many months out.

After earning the first doctoral degree ever awarded in the new field of addictive nutrition, I wrote *Potatoes Not Prozac*, which introduces the theory of sugar sensitivity and explains how food can be used to change brain and body chemistry—food in addition to medication or as an alternative to medication. The book identifies all the physical and emotional symptoms that my clients and I experienced—depression, mood swings, compulsivity, and weight issues—as evidence of sugar sensitivity. Friends told friends about sugar sensitivity and the book became a bestseller.

To provide a supportive community for *Potatoes Not Prozac* readers I designed a website (www.radiantrecovery.com). In the past two years, it has had more than 5 million hits—150,000 unique visitors—and a forum with more than 10,000 pages of letters. People from all over the world continue to tell me that the ideas in the book have changed their lives. They are thrilled with the information found on the website, but they want more—more information on what sugar addiction is and how it works; more insight on how sugar addiction is connected to sugar sensitivity; and more details on how to move out of sugar addiction. To expand our healing story to an audience of readers as well as Web users, I've written this new book.

The Sugar Addict's Total Recovery Program gives you more of what my readers have asked for . . . more of the science of sugar sensitivity introduced in *Potatoes Not Prozac* and a road map for working with your own body chemistry. This book gives you a well-tuned version of the food plan I first created for my clients and myself more than ten years ago.

Sugar addiction is a symptom of a deeper problem called sugar sensitivity. Sugar sensitivity is an inherited condition that makes you more reactive to imbalances in your body and brain chemistry that exist even prior to eating sweets. These imbalances create cravings, mood swings, erratic energy, and sugar addiction. This book will help you understand how sugar sensitivity can set up sugar addiction and make you feel crazy. It will help you:

- Understand *why* you feel the way you do
- Learn how you can fix the problem yourself—naturally
- Guide you through the process of making successful changes
- Maintain the changes you make over the long haul

The goal of this program is not to be perfect or to go off sugar for the rest of your life. The goal is to become aware of what, how, and when you eat *every day* and to be in relationship to your body. Going off sugar and white things is not like going off alcohol, drugs, or nicotine. While you may pick a day to be sugar-free and go through a period of detoxing from sugar, most likely you will not be sugar-free for the rest of your life. You will simply get better and better at the process over time. Your recovery will become a way of living as you move closer to the radiant health you deserve.

The Sugar Addict's Total Recovery Program is simple, fun, to the point, and easy to follow. It's a well-tested path to success. You will hear the voices of people just like you who have recovered from their sugar addiction. Their tips, encouragement, and great-tasting recipes will help make the healing program work for you. Concrete, specific recommendations will keep you heading in the right direction. You are not alone and you *can* heal your sugar addiction.

1

Why You Are Different

If you are a sugar addict, you can't "just say no" to ice cream, candy, soda, chocolate, or cookies. If you are a sugar addict, people have been saying "watch your calories," "exercise more," "clean up your room," "stop snacking on cookies," "stop drinking," "stop smoking," or "why don't you just _____" to you nearly all your life. You fill in the blank. The message is the same, although the content may vary.

The problem is clear. You are doing something that you don't want to be doing. But the solution isn't so clear. If you could just stop it, you would! You *can't* just say no. And the longer this helplessness goes on, the more tricks you try, the more failures you have and the more hopeless you feel. On the outside you may act cool. You might even have flip responses or pat retorts, but each time you hear the "why don't you just say no" message—even if it is subtle—you brace yourself. You ask yourself: "Why can't I get it together and take care of myself? Where is my willpower? Why aren't I like other people?" They just decide to *do* something and then they follow through. Again and again you decide, you make a commitment, you start—then your resolve fades. You get busy, you get overwhelmed, you get distracted, and your intention dissipates like the morning fog in the noonday sun.

Nancy is a sugar addict. She has vowed to give up chocolate almost every day of her life. Three days into her commitment to quit, something always happens and she reaches for a candy bar. Rosemary, who is not a sugar addict, decides that chocolate isn't good for her skin. She decides to cut it out of her diet, never buys another candy bar, isn't tempted, and doesn't think of it again. Rosemary's resolve may be inconceivable to you. Nancy feels like your sister.

When you are a sugar addict, saying no is *not* an issue of willpower. Your biochemistry has a direct effect on your behavior. Your craving and desire for sugar are profoundly affected by your brain chemistry, and even more significant, by what and when you eat.

You are a sugar addict *because* you are sugar sensitive. Sugar addiction is a primary symptom of sugar sensitivity. If you are sugar sensitive and your meals are erratic, if you skip breakfast, eat lots of sweet things, drink quarts of diet soda or eat pounds of pasta and bread, then you will be depressed, moody, erratic, volatile, forgetful, and impulsive. You may have a short fuse, a short attention span, and a reputation for being all over the place. You may have trouble with your weight, you may have an eating disorder, or you may have a problem with aggression.

It has probably not occurred to you that the food you eat could have such a dramatic effect on you. You may have figured out that sometimes you are really cranky when you haven't had your "fix." You have to go out and get a pint of your special brand of ice cream even if it's eleven o'clock at night. Your friends or parents or boss may have noticed that you have something like a split personality. Sometimes you are creative, cheerful, charming, funny, and delightful. Other times you are a royal pain in the butt and even the people who love you stay out of your way. You are a sugar addict.

When you first hear me talking about sugar addiction in this way, you may not be convinced that it is a real condition. You may not think it is possible to be addicted to something so "harmless" as sugar. Stay with me while I take you through the reasoning for my position.

Criteria for Addiction

Here are the criteria the American Psychiatric Association uses to determine addiction:

- The substance is taken in greater amounts or for a longer time than intended.
- There is a persistent desire or one or more unsuccessful attempts to cut down or control use.
- Major time is spent in seeking, using, or recovering from the effects of use.
- Frequent intoxication or withdrawal interferes with responsibilities.
- There is a decreased level of social, recreational activities due to use.
- There is continued use despite adverse consequences.
- There is a marked increase in tolerance.
- There are withdrawal symptoms.
- There is use to prevent withdrawal.

Let's reframe these criteria and see if we can create a list for sugar addiction.

• The substance is taken in greater amounts or for a longer time than intended.
Have you ever planned to have just a cookie and eaten the

whole plate? Have you ever planned to have a caramel double latte once as a celebration and found yourself going back every day? Have you ever planned to have a piece of pie and eaten the *whole thing*? Can you imagine eating half a piece of cake and leaving the rest because you just weren't hungry for it?

• There is a persistent desire or one or more unsuccessful attempts to cut down or control use.

One or more unsuccessful attempts seem sort of funny to sugar addicts. Have you ever tried to control your use? Does that question make you laugh because it seems so absurd? Have you spent most of your life since eighth grade trying to cut down or control your use of sweet things? Once you start eating sweet things, you cannot stop.

• Major time is spent in seeking, using, or recovering from the effects of use.

Do you make sure you always have a can of Coke (or even Diet Coke) on your desk? Do you make a special trip to Costco to get that *big* jar of jelly beans? Do you feel an inordinate sense of relief when your family is gone so you can eat what you want? Do you have sugar hangovers and feel cranky and irritable the day after?

• Frequent intoxication or withdrawal interferes with responsibilities.

Now at first blush, you may think that your sugar use does not affect your life. But are your bills paid on time? Is your desk cleared off? Do you double-book appointments? Are you too tired to function at three in the afternoon? Are you funny, charming, and all over the place when you eat sugar or have your soda or sweetened coffee? Look at your behavior with a different eye and you may be shocked at how true this is.

• There is a decreased level of social, recreational activities due to use.

Do you prefer to be alone so you can eat what you want, when? Do you get nervous about visiting your son's apartment because you know he doesn't have *anything* there for you to eat? Do you shy away from those friends who have given up those sweet things? Are you drawn to the people doing the "reward meal" on the Carbohydrate Addict's Diet because you know you will have company in eating what you want?

• There is continued use despite adverse consequences.

This is the ringer—continued use despite adverse consequences. You know it's bad for you, you know it's killing you, you are in despair, and you go back for more. Hits kinda close to home, yes?

• There is a marked increase in tolerance.

You need more to get the same effect. One small cookie won't cut it. You have to eat the whole box. You remember not so much the high feeling, but the feeling of relief—that the world is okay, you fit, and things will be all right. But it takes more to get you there.

• There are withdrawal symptoms.

You may not have made the connection to withdrawal per se. You may simply intuitively know that you feel better if you have a cup of tea and a piece of cake. Or you know exactly how much better you will feel once you get your supply down the hatch.

• There is use to prevent withdrawal.

You know you are cranky and will feel better if you have something sweet. Your three-year-old is having a temper tantrum because you said no to her in the grocery story. You get a soda and pop it open and she sits there being a good girl. You take a sugar break at 3:00 P.M. because you know if you don't you will be a basket case by 3:30. You know what time the edginess will start.

Sobering, isn't it? Makes you think. When you first connect with this idea of sugar addiction, it may be a little scary to you. You may find it hard to put yourself in the same class as alcoholics or heroin addicts. You may have been conditioned to think that addiction is bad and only weak-willed people are addicts or alcoholics. This book will help you understand that addiction is a chemical reality. The reason you are a sugar addict is your unique body. You respond to sugar more intensely. You hurt more in withdrawal. You feel better when you have it. The physical dependence is real. You are not a bad person; this is not a character defect. Once you start to think of yourself as having a unique brain and body chemistry, you can start on the road to recovery.

You are a sugar addict because you are sugar sensitive. Sugar addiction is a *symptom* of sugar sensitivity. If you just treat the symptom by giving up sugar, you do not heal the real problem— the biochemistry of your brain and body—and you're not likely to stay away from sugar for life. The key to long-term healing is going to the *cause* of the symptom and balancing the systems that are now out of kilter.

Sugar Sensitivity: The Three Components

Sugar sensitivity describes a collection of three different inherited problems that can have a huge impact on how you feel and how you behave. At present, sugar sensitivity is a working hypothesis that has not been scientifically proven. You can't walk into your doctor's office and say, "I want a test for sugar sensitivity." But you *can* look at your moods and behaviors and take a reasonable guess about what is going on. Your body and your symptoms will guide you in designing a food plan to restore your chemical balance and heal your addiction.

Let's take a deeper look of what's behind sugar sensitivity. Each of the components—carbohydrate sensitivity, low serotonin, and low beta-endorphin—has been studied in depth, and I want to share what science shows us about them.

Carbohydrate Sensitivity

Carbohydrate sensitivity is a term scientists developed to describe a volatile blood sugar reaction to eating carbohydrates. Generally, when a person eats carbohydrates, the blood sugar rises and the body releases a chemical called insulin. The insulin allows the cells to use the sugar in the blood as energy. As the cells use up the sugar, the amount of sugar in the blood decreases. The control of the blood sugar usually works very well. It stays in balance and keeps the blood sugar level.

If the person is sensitive to carbohydrates, the blood sugar increases more rapidly than it should; the body overreacts and produces too much insulin, which causes the blood sugar level to drop quickly. Carbohydrate sensitivity causes a rapid rise and fall in both insulin and blood sugar levels.

If you are carbohydrate sensitive, you use your fuel too quickly and get into trouble. You expect your breakfast to last. A bagel and coffee works fine for your friends with a normal body chemistry, but you crash at 10:00 A.M. and feel you could eat anything in sight. Or you might feel as if you are going to pass out. You may have diagnosed yourself as hypoglycemic and believe that you need to eat every few hours. But sugar sensitivity is not the same as hypoglycemia.

In hypoglycemia, your blood sugar level drops lower than normal. Once you eat, you are restored. If you are sugar sensitive, once you eat, you may be in bigger trouble because your blood sugar and insulin levels will continue to overreact. If you continue to eat carbohydrates, your sugar levels will spike again and you will be on the prowl in another two hours.

As your blood sugar fluctuates, your mood will fluctuate with it. When your blood sugar is rising you may feel really good, even high. And when it falls, you will feel cranky and tired. You may experience huge highs and lows throughout the day and not make the connection to your blood sugar levels.

What you eat makes a huge difference in how severe the blood sugar and insulin spikes are. Carbohydrates affect your blood sugar more than proteins and fats will. Carbohydrates that are absorbed more quickly into your bloodstream will affect you even more. Many other things can affect this volatile blood sugar as well. The amount of fiber in the carbs and the amount and type of fats you eat will also determine how greatly your blood sugar is affected. One way to measure the expected effect of certain foods is called the glycemic index, which provides indications of how much different foods can cause your blood sugar to rise. Foods low in fiber and high in sugar—doughnuts, for example—have a much higher glycemic index than foods high in fiber such as whole grains.

If you are carbohydrate sensitive, the effect of high-glycemic foods on your body will be even greater. Sugars and low-fiber carbohydrates will make the highs and lows even worse. Potatoes have been dubbed a high-glycemic food by many diet doctors. To reassure you that they're not—if eaten *with* their skins— let's learn a little science about the history of the glycemic index.

Before the 1980s, physicians and dietitians who were working with diabetic patients recommended they eat a certain number of carbohydrates, including bread, rice, potato, cereal, and similar foods. Little consideration was given to any effect that these starches might have in a diabetic's body. In 1981, David Jenkins published an article in *The American Journal of*

Clinical Nutrition describing the effects on blood sugar of certain selected starches. He gave 34 men and women 50-gram servings of different starches and measured the effect on their blood sugar. He called the results the glycemic index (GI).

The foods with the lowest GI were legumes (lentils were 29 and soybeans were 15). The highest GI went to parsnips at 97, and potatoes weighed in at 70. When measured, all the foods had been eaten alone rather than as part of a complete meal. Over the years, scientists continued to explore the usefulness of the GI.

In 1993, David Trout published a study that discussed the complexity of measuring the glycemic index. He found that a number of variables have an effect on the scores. Things like the source of the starch (legume, grain, or tuber), the species of the starch, the way it was cultivated, the cooking methods, and the degree of ripeness all contributed variation. In addition, the reduction of the starch particle size before, during, and after cooking all affected the GI. The majority of the studies (approximately two-thirds) were being done with diabetics, and no studies were being done to compare the effect of the same foods, cooked in the same way, on diabetic compared to normal individuals. No testing was done on the different ways the foods affected men and women.

In 1995, Kaye Foster-Powell published the International Tables of Glycemic Index in which she reviewed and compiled the 73 studies that had been done on the subject. Her compilation was partially funded by the Australian sugar industry. She found great variations in the effects on blood sugar of the same foods and in some cases could offer no explanation. For example, porridge (i.e., oatmeal) varied from as low as 42 to a high of 75. Significantly, she noted that as particle size decreases, the GI increases.

In fact, because the GI was developed for use in diabetic diets, it was never intended to be used in isolation. Further, as

Foster-Powell's study shows, the total amount of the carbohydrate eaten, the amount and type of fat, and the fiber content *all* affect the absorption rate and its impact on the blood sugar. For me, this indicates that while the GI can be helpful in looking at the comparative effect of different foods, it should not be the only guide you use. *The Sugar Addict's Total Recovery Program* will explain the more useful guide of eating brown things (like a potato *with* the skin) rather than white things.

Brain Chemicals

The second and third components of sugar sensitivity involve two special brain chemicals. Your brain uses chemicals called neurotransmitters to send messages from one cell to another. The levels of these chemicals profoundly affect how you feel. Your brain is designed to work best when the levels are optimal and the chemicals are all in balance. The two brain chemicals most affected by sugar sensitivity are serotonin and beta-endorphin.

Low Serotonin

Serotonin is a chemical that serves as the brakes in the brain. It is the chemical that supports just saying no. If you have low levels of serotonin, you will be impulsive—you will have a hard time saying no. Your brakes don't work right. You can't "just say no."

Because you aren't able to say no to destructive behaviors, they may become compulsive. Compulsive patterns become addiction. Once you've started, you can't stop. You have what is known as low impulse control. Low serotonin sets you up biochemically. If you are sugar sensitive, being able to say no is not so much an issue of willpower as of low serotonin levels.

If you have a low level of serotonin you may also be depressed. Your depression can be made worse by the amount of light in your environment. This condition is called seasonal affective disorder, or SAD. In the winter, you may be more depressed and more compulsive about your eating. You can't stop and you feel hopeless.

Serotonin levels significantly affect low impulse control, depression, and seasonal affective disorder. Typically the solution for low levels of serotonin has been prescription antidepressants that raise serotonin levels. Drugs such as Prozac, Zoloft, Effexor, and Paxil effectively do the job. In cases of severe clinical depression, such drugs can be lifesaving. But many times these drugs are given out as a quick and easy solution to a problem that can be better handled by changes in diet and lifestyle.

In my own clinical experience, mild to moderate depression is closely tied to diet. High sugar consumption goes hand in hand with what is generally labeled as depression. I always recommend that a client try to change his diet as the first line of defense rather than the last. The solution you will learn about in *The Sugar Addict's Total Recovery Program* is an all-natural, no-drug solution. What you eat and when you eat it can have a profound effect on your serotonin levels.

Increasing serotonin levels is a two-part process. First, you need to increase the amount of an amino acid called tryptophan that your brain uses to make serotonin. Tryptophan, like all amino acids, comes from protein. If you are eating mostly starches and sugars, your diet may be low in protein. You may not be getting the tryptophan your brain needs. Eating more protein foods on a regular basis will increase the amount of tryptophan in your blood.

However, just because there is more tryptophan in your blood, it doesn't mean it can get into your brain. Your brain is very careful about what it lets in. It has a protective shield called the blood-brain barrier to screen out things that might damage the brain. When the amino acids, including tryptophan, get up to the blood-brain barrier, they compete with each other to see who can hop across first. Unfortunately, little tryptophan usually loses. I like to think of tryptophan as the amino acid runt. The big guys (the other amino acids) walk all over him and won't let him cross.

Science brings us a wonderful solution for the problem of the runt. If you eat a food that causes a release of insulin, the insulin goes up to the blood-brain barrier and calls the big guys. It says, "Hey, guys, wanna come work out at the gym?" The insulin isn't interested in runty little tryptophan, so when the big guys go off to the gym, little Mr. Tryptophan is left by himself at the blood-brain barrier. Without competition, he hops across and sacrifices himself to the serotonin factory.

The combination of regular protein and an insulin-producing carbohydrate to increase your insulin level at a specific time does wonders for your serotonin levels. A potato seems to be the ideal food for the job of getting Mr. Tryptophan into your brain to raise the serotonin. This is why my first book was called *Potatoes Not Prozac*.

Even though my recommendations for eating will seem very simple, they are carefully thought out to give you powerful results with no side effects. As you get to know how and why your body functions, you can make more and more informed choices about the best way to deal with your own symptoms. Eating in the way I recommend can increase your serotonin levels and so decrease your impulsivity, reduce your depression, and help you say no to your sugar addiction.

Low Beta-Endorphin

The third component of sugar sensitivity is low levels of beta-endorphin. Beta-endorphin is the brain chemical that is a natural painkiller. If you have a high level of beta-endorphin, you can go out on the football field and get bashed around and keep going. If you have a low level, you cry at the drop of a hat.

When you get an endorphin rush and feel euphoric, that is beta-endorphin being activated.

Beta-endorphin levels also affect your self-esteem, your sense of confidence, your being shy, and your feeling out of the circle. If you have low levels of beta-endorphin, you can feel lonely and disenfranchised from the world. This is not merely a psychological response; it is a biochemical one.

Sugar, like heroin, alcohol, and morphine, activates beta-endorphin. Because of the beta-endorphin release, all these can make you feel euphoric. But sugar-sensitive people will feel more euphoria than others do. People who are sugar sensitive have lower levels of beta-endorphin than normal people do. The sugar-sensitive brains try to compensate for low levels of beta-endorphin by upregulating—opening more beta-endorphin receptors. Because the sugar-sensitive person is in an upregulated state, she gets a bigger hit than her normal friend does. This is why she feels she died and went to heaven after a hot fudge sundae, while her friend simply thinks it tasted good. She devours a whole bag of chocolate chip cookies; her friend can eat one bite and leave the rest. He wants six beers rather than one or the whole bottle of wine instead of one glass. Sugar sets the sugar-sensitive person up for sugar addiction.

When the sugar-sensitive person tries to stop using the sugar that evokes this wonderful beta-endorphin response, the receptors start screaming. This is called withdrawal. The person experiencing withdrawal may feel cranky, irritable, and out of sorts but never know it is last night's sugar binge creating the horrible feelings. Cravings loom large as the beta-endorphin receptors scream and relief is as close as a can of soda or a doughnut. The physical dependence on sugar to relieve the discomfort of withdrawal reinforces the need to use more and more sugar. The addiction grows into a real problem.

The Story of the C57 Mice

My excitement about beta-endorphin and its relationship to sugar addiction started from learning about and studying the work of Dr. Christine Gianoulakis at McGill University. In doing research on beta-endorphin and alcoholism, Dr. Gianoulakis found that alcoholics have lower levels of beta-endorphin than people who are not drawn to alcohol do. She also found that children and grandchildren of alcoholics are born with lower levels of beta-endorphin. This means that they are born with a genetic predisposition to alcoholism even if they do not drink. These very important findings came from many years of research working with different strains of mice in the laboratory.

Before she ever even examined people, Dr. Gianoulakis worked with two different strains of mice that responded to the effects of alcohol in very different ways. Science laboratories breed different strains of mice to have different chemistry. The C57GL/6 mice had a far more potent reaction to drinking than their "dry" brothers and sisters, the DBA/2 mice, did. Essentially, the C57s got drunker more quickly. In scientific terms, they are called alcohol-preferring mice. The DBAs are called alcohol-avoiding mice.

Dr. Gianoulakis and her colleagues wanted to determine a biochemical reason that these two strains responded so differently to alcohol. They discovered that the C57s and the DBAs have very different levels of the brain chemical beta-endorphin. The C57 mice are born with much lower levels of beta-endorphin. To compensate for this lower level, their brains increase their receptivity to beta-endorphin (upregulation), which results in a bigger response to things that evoke beta-endorphin. This explains why they have a bigger response to alcohol.

The C57 mice also have a very big interest in sugars. The C57 mice prefer the taste of sweet things far more than their buddies the DBA mice do. Sugars such as alcohol evoke beta-endorphin. So the brains of C57 mice respond to the beta-endorphin effect more intensely.

Scientists also learned that the C57 and DBA mice also respond to painkillers very differently. C57 mice have a reaction to morphine thirty-five times more powerful than that of DBA mice. Thirty-five times is a huge difference. Sugar creates a response in the brain using the same biochemical pathways as morphine, and both affect the beta-endorphin system. This explains why you as a sugar addict have a far more powerful reaction to sugar than your non-sugar-sensitive friends do.

Here are some more differences. The C57 mice get hyperactive when given morphine. DBA mice do not. Scientists have not tested whether C57 mice are more likely to be hyperactive from sugar than DBA mice are, but I speculate that they might be. When the scientists say sugar does not cause hyperactivity in children, I wonder if they are testing children who are not sugar sensitive.

When withdrawing from morphine, C57 mice become lethargic and passive. Lethargy and passivity may be very familiar responses for you as well whenever you realize you need a sugar fix and can't have one! While the little mice don't actually have couches to curl up on and wait for the pain to pass, you do. But you may never have connected these feelings to the process of beta-endorphin withdrawal.

Sugar-activated beta-endorphin changes emotions as well as physical feelings. Not only does sugar reduce physical pain in C57 mice; it also reduces the pain of loss or social isolation. When baby mice are taken from their mothers, they cry. Scientists measured the number of times the babies cried in a specified number of minutes. They gave the babies sugar water, and no surprise, they stopped crying. The "isolation distress" was significantly lessened by sugar. Sugar creates a temporary flood of beta-endorphins, thus numbing the emotional pain of separation. You may not call the pain of loneliness "isolation distress," but you know that sweet foods give you comfort and make you feel less isolated and alone.

Here is another fascinating finding about the little C57 mice. When put in a no-win situation, the DBA mice looked for an escape, while the C57 mice crouched and became immobile and defensive. Think of that. The non-sugar-sensitive strain got mobilized to find solutions, while the sugar-sensitive mice sat on the couch and argued about why they couldn't go for it.

Shift this information to people and just hear the DBAs saying to their C57 friends, "Why don't you just go get a new job if you are so unhappy? That's what I would do." Hear them ask, "Why don't you just say no?" The DBAs decide to diet and do, and then lose ten pounds in a month. They are the ones who give up chocolate for Lent and never look back, the ones who carried a little orange pumpkin at Halloween instead of a laundry bag.

The scientists doing this research have not started thinking of the C57s as a sugar-sensitive strain, but I think it is only a short step from the profile of a C57 mouse to the profile of a sugar-sensitive person. In my mind, the match is uncanny. If you start thinking of yourself as a big C57 mouse, you can have lots of clues about why you act the way you do. You will also understand why your DBA friends can't make sense of your way of being in the world.

What Does C57-ness Mean for You?

You may have felt like an "alien" if you grew up surrounded by DBAs. But now you can take comfort in the science of these mice. Just as scientists do not trash the little C57s or consider them inferior to the DBAs, you now know that the mice are simply two distinct strains with two very different body chemistries.

There is no right or wrong mouse. No good or bad one. No good body type or bad body type.

The scientific dispassion about mouse strains can teach you compassion for yourself in your own journey to healing. When you look at the C57s' tendencies as just another way of being, you open yourself to compassion for your way of being in the world. And as you learn how your sugar-sensitive body works, you can start making choices for healing.

Think of yourself as the human equivalent of a C57. You love sweets. You are comforted by sugars. You turn to sugar for solace when you feel isolated. It gives you courage when you are afraid and takes away the pain when you are hurting. Sweet foods can give you "motor mouth." You become engaging, funny, and self-confident. Sometimes your friends wonder if you have been drinking. Often, you choose other C57s as friends, so you go out for coffee and have cake instead and really enjoy your social times. Having coffee with your cake feels like heaven. You get clear, focused, and relaxed for about thirty minutes. You love that feeling. Your DBA friends actually enjoy the *coffee* and care less about the sweets you always have with it.

When you try to go off sugar you sit around and wait till the discomfort passes. You crouch like the C57s. You hunker down with your discomfort. You go immobile. You feel as if your cells are made of lead and are screaming. You feel the effect of withdrawal in your gut, your skin, and your brain—wherever there are beta-endorphin receptor sites. You get so uncomfortable, you go back to the food that comforts you. You know that sweet foods give you energy. You don't realize that the sugar is resolving the lethargy of beta-endorphin withdrawal.

When you feel defeated and overwhelmed, you go into what I call "the great sleep"—lying on the couch and not moving. Or you may act as a hero and never appear defeated at all. Outwardly, you encourage everyone else to believe that you are absolutely in control. But inside, you are holding on by a thread and feel horrible. When faced with the same crises you find yourself in, your DBA friends get energized. Yet you feel inadequate and overwhelmed. You take Prozac; they change jobs and get a promotion. You hate this injustice and have not had a clue how biochemically mediated it is.

Being sugar sensitive is very confusing because alcohol, sugar, and white things get you mobilized, make you brave, funny, and self-confident. You may not have noticed that this energy lasts for only a little while. When the beta-endorphin hit wears off, you crash. You go into withdrawal, which is very uncomfortable. You become even more immobile, hopeless, demoralized, overwhelmed, and tearful, but you do not make the connection to withdrawal. What you do remember is that when you use sugar, you feel okay. So you are willing to trade thirty minutes, then twenty minutes, then ten minutes of feeling okay for the rest being horrible because you are so desperate to feel okay. You will do anything not to experience the pain of sugar withdrawal.

This is why so many people who write to me lament that they cannot imagine giving up sugar. It's the only thing that makes life worth living. Now, thinking rationally, we both know that sugar is not the thing making life manageable. Yet I hear this all the time. This is sugar addiction. This is being caught in a place that is killing you, but you have no idea what is really going on. But don't feel bad about this. You *can't* see what's going on when you are in the middle of it.

Ironically, many sugar-sensitive people are very intolerant of alcoholics and drug addicts. They do not realize that sugar addiction is affecting them in the same way. Alcoholism and drug addiction are only more intense forms of sugar addiction. Addiction creates a life driven by the desperate need to feel better and to escape the terror of the withdrawal, and a life centered on getting your fix.

The Sugar Addict's Total Recovery Program gives you a name for what is happening. It provides a vocabulary and concepts to explain your behavior. Suddenly, your feelings start to make sense. The vague knowing you have had for a while (sugar sensitives are intuitive people!) gets a name. You don't have to think of yourself as hopeless, depressed, and out of control. Your inherited biochemistry is the culprit, not laziness, lack of discipline, or mental illness.

Remember to think of yourself as a big C57 mouse so that you can connect with what these mouse studies mean for you. Those things that you have considered character flaws for all this time are a function of your sugar-sensitive biochemistry. You believe (erroneously) that DBA behavior is good and C57 behavior is bad. Society tends to recognize and value DBA behavior as the standard for being good, so, picking up on that attitude, you have usually judged yourself harshly. It is time to change your sense of who you are.

Sex Differences in Brain Chemicals

Men generally have higher levels of both serotonin and beta-endorphin than women do. This difference in brain chemicals can shed some light on why men on the whole are less impulsive and have a higher tolerance for pain than women do. However, some men (children and grandchildren of alcoholics) inherit lower levels of both serotonin and beta-endorphin. Their levels are more like those of women.

These are the sugar-sensitive men. They may be seen as sensitive guys because they are more aware of feelings and more vulnerable to both physical and emotional pain. Sometimes this vulnerability creates a great deal of pain in childhood for these men. I used to ask the male clients in my clinic whether any of them had been called a sissy as a child. One hundred percent answered yes. These men were all alcoholics and all sugar sensitive. They were more likely to have trouble with impulse control. They would get angry and shoot off their mouths. They would drink (which reduced their impulse control even more) and then would shoot off more than their mouths.

What I saw in the clinic with alcoholic men is now mirrored with what I see in sugar-sensitive men doing this program. The similarities are striking. Sugar-sensitive men can be moody, introverted, and intuitive. Their creativity and humor about being sensitive may mask deep feelings of inadequacy and low self-esteem. They may also mask these feelings by being alcoholic, abusive, angry, and out of control. Or they may simply be depressed and turn to alcohol for solace.

Because the feelings that come from low levels of serotonin and beta-endorphin are so hard to manage, sugar-sensitive people continue to be drawn to the substances that seem to make them feel better. The "feel better" substances are alcohol, drugs, and sugar. Often sugar-sensitive men will be drawn to alcohol as the solution and sugar-sensitive women will be drawn to sugar as the solution. Both affect the same biochemical vulnerability caused by low beta-endorphin.

Because women are born with naturally lower levels of beta-endorphin and serotonin than men, they are more likely to be impulsive and depressed and to have lower self-esteem. Women who are children or grandchildren of alcoholics will have even lower levels of beta-endorphin. Women's levels also fluctuate each month in sync with the menstrual cycle. Beta-endorphin for women peaks at ovulation and then drops precipitously before menstruation. The fluctuations in beta-endorphin correspond with PMS symptoms. PMS brings not only physical symptoms but also feelings of hopelessness, inadequacy, and a desire to isolate yourself; this is due to dropping beta-endorphin levels. Many report food cravings during this time that seem impossible to resist.

In addition, with the onset of perimenopause or menopause, the peaking of beta-endorphin around ovulation diminishes and women may find themselves in a biochemical crisis. The changed levels of beta-endorphin add to an already complex hormonal shift. They may feel even more drawn to substances that evoke beta-endorphin—sugar and alcohol and chocolate.

Women who are the children of alcoholics are even more at risk. They start off with lower levels of beta-endorphin and can be in big trouble in the second phase of their menstrual cycles because their beta-endorphin levels drop even further. They may experience severe PMS or feel increasingly depressed or inadequate, even though rationally they know these feelings arc not warranted. Cravings for carbohydrates, chocolates, or sweets may increase dramatically. These cravings are chemical. Low beta-endorphin means low self-esteem and cravings. The chocolate response and the sugar addiction come out of the biochemistry of sugar sensitivity.

The Three-Legged Stool

Let's put the three parts together: carbohydrate sensitivity causing volatile blood sugar, low serotonin, and low beta-endorphin. Sugar sensitivity involves each of the three parts, but it is also affected by the relationship of these parts. Imagine a three-legged stool with blood sugar (BS), serotonin (5HT), and beta-endorphin (BE) each acting as a leg. A deficit in any or all three of the legs makes the stool off balance. Anyone who tries to sit or stand on it will fall.

Each sugar-sensitive person may have problems with a different leg of the stool. Sugar-sensitive people with deficits in blood sugar (BS) will be volatile and moody; sugar-sensitive people with low levels of serotonin (5HT) will be depressed and impulsive; and sugar-sensitive people with low beta-endorphin (BE) will have low self-esteem, feel socially isolated, and have a very low tolerance for painful situations. Sugar-sensitive people with deficits in more than one area would have the symptoms of both—or all three—areas.

Not only are there symptoms associated with each leg of the stool, there appear to be unique dietary habits associated with each. The BSs are likely to skip meals, forget breakfast, and eat erratically. They suddenly realize they are desperately hungry and grab anything they can find. The 5HTs are drawn to sweets, bread, and pasta—their comfort foods. They tend to be binge eaters or compulsive eaters and often struggle with their weight. When lack of impulse control and compulsive eating combine, the result is often serious weight gain.

The BEs are hard-line sugar and alcohol lovers. These are the ones who play with the edge, flirting with danger and squeaking by. They are the miracle workers who push deadlines and come through in a crunch, no matter the cost to their bodies. The BEs may be normal-weight men and women who are closet sugar users. They may be nervous, energetic adrenaline junkies who take great pride in not eating. When they do eat, they grab white carbohydrates and sugars to go with their third cup of coffee. Because they may not have weight problems, it is hard for them to connect with the seriousness of their sugar sensitivity or sugar addiction.

Working with All Three

Most of my own clients seem to be a combination of all three: volatile blood sugar (BE), serotonin (5HT) and beta-endorphin (BE). They get to check the box marked "all of the above." They are sugar addicts because they are sugar sensitive. Sugar sensitivity is a very complicated problem. Until now, solutions have targeted only one leg of the stool at a time. Trying to figure out which leg of the stool to treat and then figuring out the degree of deficit has been difficult for doctors to sort out. Few doctors understand the relationship of all three parts of the stool, making it even harder for you to find a solution.

When you most need a solution, when you are most unbalanced, you are the least able to sort out the answer. You may not have a clue about why you feel so bad, so you settle for the first advice you are given. In good faith, you seek help and are told to do what the doctor orders. The most likely solution is a prescription for an antidepressant. The antidepressants work with only the serotonin leg of the stool. Unfortunately, drugs can be hit-or-miss, and they don't always work or keep working. The dosage needs to be adjusted. The brand needs to be changed. The depression may get better, but then it comes back. The problem remains, and the side effects are difficult. You lose weight and then regain it. You have no sex drive. You are still tired. You still have mood swings, and they are getting worse. Only now, you feel despondent because you have spent so much time, money, and energy on healing. You *should* be fixed. But the other legs of the stool are still imbalanced. Low beta-endorphin hasn't been touched by any of the interventions you've tried. Your blood sugar levels still fluctuate wildly.

Because of your weight gain, you intuitively feel that if you found the right diet and lost weight, you would feel better. But until now, most of the diets, like the drugs you have tried, target only one or two of the legs of the stool. They offer you hope, and in fact work well in addressing one piece. But they are not complete.

You may feel a sense of hope as you read this book. You may feel that if you simply go off of sugar, you will be okay. **But you cannot treat your sugar addiction by simply going off sugar.** You need to treat your underlying sugar sensitivity and heal the imbalance that creates your continuing need to use sugar addictively. You need to restore all three legs of the stool. The story is far bigger than learning to "just say no." *The Sugar*

Addict's Total Recovery Program will address all three problems contributing to your addiction and give you a solution that will finally work.

Why Other Eating Plans Haven't Worked for Sugar Addicts

Now that you have a better understanding of how blood sugar, serotonin, and beta-endorphin are so important to the sugar-sensitive person who is sugar addicted, let's take a look at some of the dietary plans you may have tried. Look at them through the filter of this new information to understand why they worked or didn't work for you.

The Atkins Plan

Robert Atkins in *Dr. Robert Atkins' New Diet Revolution* suggests shifting to a low-carbohydrate, high-protein, and high-fat diet. Atkins says carbs are bad because they produce insulin, and his plan is very appealing. You can have steak, bacon, cheese, eggs, butter, and cream. Staying away from desserts doesn't seem so bad in the face of the comfort of fat. And, most important to many of us, the Atkins plan promises dramatic results quickly. You lose weight. You lose weight fast. And you seem to feel terrific . . . for a while.

Atkins is right about sugar and simple carbohydrates creating weight gain, but he makes no allowance for sugar sensitivity and addiction. Just start the diet, stay on it, he says, and you will feel better. But if a sugar sensitive adheres to the Atkins plan, she will have a problem in her serotonin and beta-endorphin production. If she follows Atkins to the letter, she will minimize her insulin production. But her body *requires* insulin to move tryptophan from her bloodstream into her brain *to make serotonin.* If the insulin response is minimized dramatically, the serotonin level drops and the ability to "just say no" will drop dramatically. She will become depressed.

Six or eight weeks into the Atkins plan, a sugar addict will be one cranky puppy. If she tries a little something sweet, her beta-endorphin cravings will awaken. The sleeping giant of sugar addiction, now roused, will take her to the bakery, the ice cream store, or the bar. She will feel wonderful with the "just a little" something, truly mellow, relaxed, hopeful, and peaceful. So "just a little" more will seem fine. Two weeks later, she will discover she is in a full-blown relapse. And she won't be able to stop. Her impulse control mechanism, which is dependent upon serotonin, will have been shot. This is called rebound, and she is in big trouble.

Trying Out the Zone and Protein Power

The Zone is more tempered in its instructions. "Balance," Barry Sears says. "Seek balance." The formula 30-40-30 became a key word for Zone dieters as many worked hard to get Sears's ratios down at each meal. Mastery of the formula promises a slim body and high energy forever. But sugar-sensitive dieters often drift away from the rigor Sears demands. Sears also says the 30 percent carbohydrates could be jelly beans or white bagels. Even his special Zone bars have sugar in them. Sugar-sensitive dieters find themselves eating five or six bars a day and wondering why the plan isn't working. While the Zone plan does offer a masterful response to altering insulin levels and hormonal levels, it does not address addiction or beta-endorphin priming. Its very design is to reduce insulin action that over time reduces the availability of tryptophan for conversion into serotonin. It's no surprise that many sugar-sensitive people fall from the Zone within a few weeks.

The *Protein Power* diet seems more promising for sugar addicts and sugar-sensitive people. Like Atkins, Michael and Mary Dan Eades talk about the need to control insulin levels by shifting away from carbohydrates and moving toward protein and fat. *Protein Power* seems kinder and more sensible than Atkins.

While promising dramatic results, it offers a workable plan. Protein Power dieters felt better, lost weight, and kept working at it. But something was missing. Six to eight weeks into the plan, sugar sensitives started getting restless, noticing carbohydrates wherever they went. Bagels and muffins started calling to them again. Many sugar sensitives slipped, had a few servings of a favorite comfort food—and found themselves sliding into bread, cookies, or ice cream. They couldn't understand why they had fallen off the program so quickly.

The Protein Power diet does leave sugar sensitives less vulnerable to failure than the Atkins plan, but it doesn't deal with either addiction or the brain functions affected by diet. The balanced approach to nutrition in *Protein Power* is healthier and more reasonable, and keeping the fat level at 30 percent protects dieters from fat-induced insulin resistance. But the Zone, Protein Power, and Atkins plans, when followed carefully, will contribute to a problematic drop in serotonin. The clarity and focus dieters feel for six to eight weeks on the plan dissipate. The diet starts to seem too restrictive, and once more sugar sensitives are on the prowl for something to eat that will make them feel better. This restlessness and irritability is low serotonin speaking, not a lack of willpower. With low serotonin you and your diet are in trouble.

The Hellers' Plan

Richard and Rachael Heller's *The Carbohydrate Addict's Diet* taps into many dieters' intuition that something more is going on for them in their biochemistry than for other dieters. The term "carbohydrate addict" sounds on target. Many people *know* they feel like addicts—helpless and out of control—around carbs or sweets.

The Hellers expand on the important role of insulin in losing weight. They promise that if you have your carbs in a particular way and at a particular time of day, you can eat whatever you want. Their idea of a "reward meal" is thrilling to dieters who are also sugar sensitive and sugar addicts. Dieters know they can do anything they have to during the day if at 6:10 P.M. they can get bread, wine, pasta, and ice cream as their reward.

The Hellers also promise that this reward meal will help to take care of serotonin levels, which control feeling full. The reward meal raises your serotonin, thus quieting your cravings and controlling your addiction. This is an awesome promise. Pay attention, be rigorous all day, then get a "reward." You have only to wait until evening and then you will be fine. And you will lose weight, feel great, and never have to diet again.

However, the "reward meal" is a ticket to disaster for sugar addicts and sensitives. It reinforces the core of addictive thinking by reinforcing the idea of cutting a deal and just hanging on until the reward time rolls around. The deal is being able to have anything you want if you have it within a certain time window. But when you choose your favorite reward foods, sweets and white flour breads, you are priming your beta-endorphin level. You will activate cravings leading your brain and body to expect—in fact, to *demand*—more of the same. So the very thing you believe is the source of your comfort (the reward) is actually feeding your addiction to sugars and carbs and reinforcing your cravings.

The addictive tendency of a sugar or carbohydrate addict's biochemistry is *not* due to low serotonin, but to beta-endorphin. The Hellers' reward meal boosts a sugar addict's beta-endorphin level temporarily; a short while later, it sets off cravings. Eventually, she slips off the plan. First, her reward meal may continue beyond the allotted hour. Then the reward becomes a binge. Three weeks later, she may wake up in shame, horror, and confusion. She has gained weight. She is out of control once again. She doesn't know what happened. Her beta-endorphin system got dramatically out of balance.

Sugar Busters!

Sugar Busters! is straightforward. "Just say no to sugar," the authors say, reinforcing the message that sugar addicts and sensitives have heard all their life. The authors write that all foods made with sugar and white flour are bad, so stop eating bad stuff. But many sugar sensitives and addicts developed headaches, irritability, and serious crankiness on the Sugar Busters! program. Their withdrawal was too quick and too intense. The diet had no support to increase serotonin. Nor does the plan deal with addiction. "Just say no" doesn't work for most sugar sensitives and addicts.

Looking at these different weight-loss diets together, it is easy to see that none of them addresses all the components of sugar sensitivity. The needs of all three systems—carbohydrate sensitivity that creates blood sugar volatility, serotonin, and beta-endorphin—have to be addressed or you will continue your lifelong struggle with food cravings and addiction.

2

The Solution

The Sugar Addict's Total Recovery Program works with all three biochemical components of the sugar-sensitive brain and body to heal sugar sensitivity and addiction. This recovery plan very simply says, "Let's get to the heart of the problem. Let's heal the conditions that make you fat, make you impulsive, and make you crazy. The solution is not *no* carb, but *slow* carb. Slow carbs contain whole grains and a lot of fiber. Not high protein, but regular and sufficient protein." The plan provides a way to reduce your insulin overall but retain a timed response to increase your serotonin, to minimize your cravings by stopping the beta-endorphin priming, and to increase your beta-endorphin production.

The Sugar Addict's Total Recovery Program is a long-range solution, not a quick fix. The plan tells you what to do based on your brain and body chemistry and explains why you are the way you are. It teaches you what being sugar sensitive means and shows you what you can do about it starting right away, today. It also takes the radical approach that you don't need to follow a rigid program to free yourself from sugar addiction. Designing your own plan, knowing your own style, and getting to know your own body with its unique reactions is an approach totally different from those of most popular diet plans.

You need a solution that works for you, a simple solution that you can understand and implement. You are ready to get healthy and feel better. Here is where the food plan comes in. The food plan addresses all three problems at once without side effects and at no cost. It stabilizes your blood sugar, raises serotonin, and reduces the overreaction of beta-endorphin to sweet foods that creates cravings. The final part of the plan is designed to enhance your everyday level of beta-endorphin.

Because the plan is so manageable, you can focus on doing the food without having to measure, balance, calculate, and adjust for each deficit. In essence, you do the food and the plan takes care of the healing. The process accounts for what seems to be the miraculous change users have reported.

Introducing the Seven Steps

I will talk about the seven steps of the plan in more detail in the next chapters, but here it is important for you to see how the steps fit with the science. Step 1 (eating breakfast with protein) stabilizes your blood sugar and sets up having enough tryptophan in your blood to manufacture serotonin. Step 2 (journaling) teaches you how to read your body and adjust the rhythm and pace to your own needs. Step 2 also teaches you to see which of the three legs of your biochemical stool is most off balance. Step 3 (three meals a day with protein) stabilizes your blood sugar further and prepares for the increase of serotonin production.

Step 4 (having the vitamins and the nightly potato) increases your serotonin and gives your brain what it needs to manufacture serotonin. Step 5 (shifting from whites to browns) moves you away from your love affair with carbohydrates. It gives your body the positive effect of carbohydrates while eliminating the part that creates craving. Step 6 (taking out the sugar) reduces the craving for sugar by eliminating beta-endorphin priming. Eliminating the priming heals the addiction. Step 7 (finding radiance, or simply getting a life) teaches you the behaviors that enhance the increase of beta-endorphin.

The seven steps work their magic. You get a biochemical body-brain stool with three solid legs. You don't have to figure out a complex healing prescription; you just do the food, listen to your body, and make the adjustments to heal your own sugar sensitivity and addiction. You, not some outside expert, prescribe what is right for you. Whether you are male or female, whether you are fat or thin, whether you are depressed or addictive doesn't matter. The starting food plan is the same for all. The refinements come as you learn your body and your needs. Simplicity makes it work.

There are also seven steps in my first book, *Potatoes Not Prozac*, but the steps in the Sugar Addict's Total Recovery Program are a little different from the way they were first written. I originally recommended starting with the food journal. For some people, however, even that was too hard. I want you to have confidence that you can do this plan. Now I recommend starting with breakfast.

Here are the steps:

1. Eat breakfast with protein.
2. Journal what you eat and how you feel.
3. Eat three meals a day with protein.
4. Take the recommended vitamins and have a potato before bed.
5. Shift from white foods to brown foods.
6. Reduce or eliminate sugars.
7. Create a new life.

I will say more about each step as we move through the book. The steps may seem ridiculously simple to you. They are simple, but a bit harder to do than you may think. Notice that going off sugar is Step 6, not Step 1. This entire book is aimed at getting you to go slow and follow the steps in order.

Why the Steps Are in This Order

If you try to do this program without following the steps in the order presented, the program won't work for you. It's that simple. You may feel worse instead of better and decide to give up because the "program doesn't work."

If you can trust that there is a method to my madness, and do the steps in the order recommended, you will stabilize each of the biochemical functions involved in your sugar sensitivity and addiction. We will stabilize your blood sugar, increase your serotonin, reduce the beta-endorphin priming, and then increase your beta-endorphin levels.

Later on, you'll have plenty of room to exercise your own judgment and make your own choices—you'll tailor the details of the plan to suit you. But don't tinker with the big picture. And don't rush to the end. You do not need to be dramatic and do it all at once. If you try to go off sugar, alcohol, drugs, and white flour—even caffeine and nicotine, for example—you will feel terrible. Your head will hurt and you will get both irritable and panicky. Don't do it that way. Quiet your sugar-driven impatience and follow the steps.

Do the steps in the sequence, and you will get wonderful results. That is my promise to you.

Don't Rush to the End

"Okay," you might be saying. "I'll do the steps in order, but I'll do them one right after the other. Let's get on with this. If this works, I want to heal this problem NOW!" This is your sugar sensitivity talking. Your sugar-sensitive brain, with its love of impulsivity, wants you to do everything right away. "Give it to me all at once," it says.

Please don't do it!

Do one step at time. Do not proceed to the next step until you have mastered the one before it. Start with breakfast with protein. The steps need to go in sequence. Each step builds on the previous one. The food plan is designed to change your blood chemistry and improve your neurotransmitter function. It will stabilize your blood sugar level so your moods don't swing from extreme (and often unrealistic) optimism to despair. It will increase your serotonin level so you have more impulse control and are less depressed. Finally, it will optimize your beta-endorphin level so your self-esteem increases and your interest in sweets evaporates. The food plan will create changes way beyond anything you have imagined. This plan heals more of your life than just your sugar sensitivity and addiction.

So even though the steps may seem obvious and simplistic, they actually create profound physical and emotional change. Give your body (and your sugar-sensitive brain) time to get used to each change before going on to the next step.

The key to success with this program is to go slowly and go in sequence.

Getting Ready to Start

As you get ready to start, you may have different feelings depending on what sex you are. Men and women seem to have very different styles in doing the program. Often, the guys will write me a short note and say, "Okay, tell me what to do, Coach." I give them the steps and they go off and do them—and they tend to do them quite well the first time out.

Then one of two things happens. I hear from the first type a year later. They report that the plan made a significant positive change in their lives and that is the last I hear from them. Often these are guys who are also recovering alcoholics. They have done twelve-step work and the food plan simply completes their program.

The second type also does the program really well initially. Then, about three months into it, they discover all sorts of unexpected feelings. And they are spooked big-time. Their food gets wobbly; they get confused and come back to start at the beginning. Eventually, as they learn to manage their new feelings, they do fine.

Women, on the other hand, often fuss for several months before actually starting. They talk about their ambivalence, about feelings, about fear and confusion. They don't want to give up their good friend Mr. Chocolate; they often go out on a "last" sugar run, which of course exaggerates everything they are feeling. And then they quietly start with the program by eating breakfast with protein every day. Their feelings become manageable, and they get back to the plan.

Whether your feelings come before you start or several months into the program, pay attention to them, notice them, record them in your journal, but do not get distracted by them. Simply focus on the food and use the feelings to guide your progress and you will be more successful. You do not have to understand or make sense of all the feelings for the program to work. You simply want to learn the connections between your moods and what you are eating.

Notice your ambivalence if it comes up, write about it in your food journal, and keep doing the food. There is no one right way to do the plan. Learn your own style and rhythm of making change so you can tailor your plan to work for you.

Sugar Feelings

When sugar-sensitive people first learn about their body chemistry, they generally feel a great sense of relief. They feel as if they have finally "come home" to a story that makes sense and puts the pieces together. They want to rush into doing the whole program at once. You may feel this as well.

Even though you feel excited to have found something that sounds so right on, you may also be afraid that it won't really work. You may be terrified that you are being set up to hope only to fail once again. You want to do it all, and you are terrified that you will have to give up what comforts you. You may have a love/hate reaction to these ideas. And your feelings about giving up sugar may be so intense that they spook you.

Tips from the Field: You Are Not Alone

Here are some of the things that run through people's heads before they start the program.

- **Will this really work for me?**
- **Will it help the depression?**
- **How will I remember all the details?**
- **How will I keep a journal?**
- **Does this mean I'm going to have to cook?** (I can't cook. I know how, but I am blocked. I can't seem to ever get my kitchen cleaned up enough to cook in there. And if I cook, I'll have to clean up.)

Your enthusiasm and fear are filtered through what I call sugar feelings. Sugar feelings come from an unbalanced biochemistry and the foods you are now eating. Sugar feelings distort the natural reactions you have. Sugar feelings make things seem bigger, more dramatic, more exciting—and scarier. Whenever you feel scared or doubtful, simply take a deep breath, have a cup of tea, and sit with the feelings. Be patient with yourself. Do nothing. Do *not* start changing all your food right away. Just keep reading, reflecting, and tempering your desire to do everything right now. Do one step, one choice at a time.

Keeping Things Simple

It is easy for you to get overwhelmed when you are presented with lots of new information. That's actually a symptom of sugar sensitivity.

My job is to keep things simple, to get you started on this program without overwhelming you with information. The early part of your journey will be more directive and specific. You will have options, but the basic steps you will need to take will be described clearly. These changes will set up your body for success with the rest of this program. These very first steps you take will begin healing your sugar sensitivity—which will make doing the rest of this program easier.

The Sugar Addict's Total Recovery Program includes the experience and expertise of the people who have been working the program over the last few years. As you may know from your own experience, sugar-sensitive people are gifted and creative, with a lot to say. The Web site has hosted exchanges that have tested this material in an active community. I have read more than 40,000 letters on the subjects we will be discussing in this book. *The Sugar Addict's Total Recovery Program* will give you the nuts-and-bolts guidance continually being refined on the Web by people who used to feel just as you do now, but who now live free of cravings and mood swings.

Here is an email from someone who has been sending her questions and comments to the Web site regularly:

I've been part of this community for more than a year. I think I was among the first to check it out when it got started. You wouldn't have recognized any of us back then!

The forum is so many things to me. It is a refuge, it is a library, it is a friend, it is an awakening, it is a barometer, it is a sounding board, it is a course correction, it is ideas, it is progress. . . .

I wouldn't have stayed on the journey without this community! Yet I've almost walked away several times because the pain this process would tap into was too intense. But something would happen EVERY TIME I thought of leaving that would keep me here. Somehow the support and encouragement I needed would come through.

I LOVE what this community is. I've never experienced anything like it. Thank you for being a part of my healing.

The Sugar Addict's Total Recovery Program will take you through the seven steps one at a time. But it will also give you practical tips and advice to help you do the program. You will learn

- What to order in restaurants
- What to cross off your grocery list
- What you can fix quickly for dinner
- What to eat when you have sugar cravings
- Why potatoes are good for you
- How to make friends with veggies
- How to get back on the plan when you've slipped

You will also share recipes, shopping lists, and tips for coping with tough situations, such as a business meeting that runs past your usual mealtime. This book puts the answers to all these questions—and more—in one place.

Tips from the Field: Reaching Radiance

The thing that is different about me now is the way I feel. In my first couple of months on the program, I felt better outside: calmer, less nervous and shaky. Now, after four and a half months, I feel better inside: more hopeful, more excited about life, more capable, more solid, clearer, stronger. I know this is the result of a balanced brain chemistry.

—D.

Because people just like you have tested so much of what is in the Sugar Addict's Recovery Program, I know that I am giving you what you need to hear when you need to hear it. The healing process is gradual and developmental. The kind of advice you need when you first start the program is different from that you will need four months or a year later. Your brain and body will change over time. At first you may need more structure. Often people talk about the "sugar fog" they are in when they first get started. Your feelings and reactions may be colored by your sugar intake or by not eating breakfast. You may go back and forth between feeling overwhelmed by the ideas in the program and feeling wildly enthusiastic about finding an answer to your mood swings and low self-esteem.

This book is quite directive at the beginning until you are able to know and adapt to your own healing style. As you become more experienced, it will encourage you to listen to your body, understand your own rhythms, listen to your colleagues along the way, and create what works for you. The program starts by stabilizing your volatile blood sugar reactions. You will learn to eat regularly and on time. You will learn to be steady, steady, steady. You will learn to hold on through what may feel like a rather tame beginning. Next, it helps raise your serotonin levels. You will have a potato at night and experience the science behind the program right in your own body. You will also see why eating protein at each meal sets the stage for your body to make serotonin. And you will feel better almost immediately.

You will be thrilled and excited when you master the moods that have haunted you for so long. You will become more reflective and less impulsive. Rather than responding to problems or roadblocks with tears, you will start anticipating and solving problems. Even the way you think of yourself will change. If you thought you were "naturally" intense and moody, you may discover that you *are* naturally intuitive and perceptive, but not nearly as moody as you thought.

You will stop craving sugar and breads all day long. You will no longer wake up feeling hungover in the morning. You will be less cranky, less reactive. Life will seem brighter and you will be able to get to the things you have put off for years. *All* these things change as you change your food! *The Sugar Addict's Total Recovery Program* will guide you as you go.

The Best Way to Use This Recovery Program

This book is called a recovery program because it does more than simply address or cover up the symptoms of sugar sensitivity. It heals the underlying problem that causes the symptoms. But to make it work best for you, you will need to make it your own. Personalize your program so that it fits your needs, your style, and your interests.

Before you actually start the steps, here are some ideas on ways to use your book and make it into your own program.

Colored Markers—Using Yellow and Other Colors

Go to the stationery store and buy yourself several different colors of highlighter pens—maybe yellow, pink, and blue. Then, as you read the pages in this book, highlight with yellow (or whichever color you choose) the phrases and sentences that really speak to you: things you want to remember, insights that fit for you, and so on. For example, when you come to the section of Chapter 6 about planning your food, you might want to highlight in yellow the style that best describes you. You could use pink to highlight action steps you want to take, such as buying protein powder or digging out your old Crock-Pot. And you might use blue highlighter to mark the parts of the book that will help you when you're feeling cranky or having cravings.

I like yellow as a highlighter. My brain is now trained to see yellow as the code to pay attention. My books are color coded for my own style and preferences. Your book needs to reflect your style and your process.

Post-it Notes

Pepper your copy of this book with Post-it notes marking sections that you will want to refer to later, like "Ten Breakfast Ideas" or "Snacks You Can Buy at a Convenience Store." You can write the name of the section you are marking on the part of the Post-it that sticks out—it's sort of like making your own tabs to help you turn quickly to parts of the book that you will use often. You can also use the Index for guidelines.

Flags

Another trick for personalizing your book is to mark important points or sections with Post-it tape flags. You might, for example, use red flags to mark pages that have your pink-highlighted action steps, or blue flags to help you find the blue-highlighted paragraphs on coping with cravings. Or use purple tape flags to mark the sections you can turn to when you need inspiration or fellowship, such as one or more of the stories from others working the *Potatoes Not Prozac* plan.

If you want, you can write yourself a little note on the flags in

pencil or ballpoint pen (felt-tip markers won't work). Just be
sure to use the nonglossy side of the tape flag.

Writing in the Margins

Is this starting to make sense? Use the book the way I hope you
will use the food plan. Make it your own. See what works best
for you, then do the plan (and mark your book) that way. Let's
take it one step further.

As you read, make notes for yourself in the margins. Write
down any questions that you have, any personal insights that
you get, any comments you have on what you are reading. *Interact* with this book. Add your thoughts and ideas to mine. Argue
with my ideas. Test the principles of the program. Record your
reactions to the tips and action steps. Make this *your* book,
not mine.

If you don't like to write in your books, think of *The Sugar Addict's Total Recovery Program* as a workbook, the kind of book that
is *designed* to be written in.

Setting Up Your Own Notebook

If you like to keep your books clean, you can photocopy the
pages of your personal copy of *The Sugar Addict's Total Recovery
Program* that have information or advice that is important to
you. Then work with and highlight your photocopied pages.
Put the pages in a notebook that will become your own working
version of the book.

You can divide the notebook into sections that make sense to
you. Instead of making dividers labeled "Chapter 1" and "Chapter 2," maybe use "Good Ideas to Try," "Key Points," "Inspiration," and "Recipes."

One advantage of making your own notebook is that you can
add material that isn't in the book, such as printouts of the postings on our online Community Forum or recipes you find in

other books or magazines. Some people mark their own books *and* set up a notebook. But either way, make the book yours. Put it to work for you. It will be your most valuable companion on your journey from sugar sensitivity to radiance.

Tips from the Field: Slow Down

Many folks doing this program suffer from the same syndrome: trying to do too much too fast. It is really a form of sabotage. Even if it is from overeagerness, not self-destructiveness, it still rips the rug out from under every effort you make. Work the steps at the pace it takes for you to be able to stick to them. It is okay to be where you are—overweight, depressed, addicted, whatever. Where you are is where you start.

—D.

3

Getting Started:
Steps 1 and 2

Now that you have been playing with your book a bit, let's actually get started with your program. The first step is to eat breakfast with protein every day.

Step 1. Eat Breakfast with Protein Every Day

Some people believe that my direction to eat breakfast every day and make sure it has protein in it is too simple. They don't think it can be part of the diet and the food plan. But this step is *hard*. It may take you months to master. Breakfast with protein . . . every day.

Don't worry about going off sugar or caffeine right now. Have French toast with sausage and a cup of espresso if you want. The sausage will be your protein. Have two scrambled eggs and juice. The eggs will be your protein. Have lox and cream cheese on a bagel. The lox (and to some extent the cream cheese) will be your protein.

Why Is Breakfast a Must?

Sugar-sensitive people are notorious for not eating breakfast. My readers have said they don't like breakfast, they aren't hungry in the morning, and even the idea of eating seems horrible.

Sugar-sensitive people sometimes do seem to feel better without breakfast. That's because when they don't eat for eight or ten hours, their body thinks they are moving toward starvation mode and releases beta-endorphin to protect them. Sugar-sensitive people are more sensitive to the (temporary) euphoric and confidence-building effects of beta-endorphin. They will often not eat because it actually *feels* better. It makes them feel strong and lean. But the beta-endorphin release masks their dropping blood sugar level. This is why they crash big time at 10 A.M. and then eat anything (usually something sweet) in sight.

I want to protect your body from the stress of the crash. I also want to help you move away from using not eating as a way of feeling beta-endorphin-induced confidence. There are healthier ways to achieve higher beta-endorphin.

Just eat breakfast with protein every morning. If you can't stand the thought of breakfast foods, eat a lunch-type meal instead. Have miso or wonton soup (the kind with chicken and shrimp added). Have corned beef hash. Have a grilled cheese sandwich. Have a burrito or chili. Have pizza (but be sure it has protein—meat or lots of cheese—on it).

Many former breakfast haters on this program started out by having a Smoothie-like George's Shake for breakfast. Use the recipe that follows, make up one of your own, or order the mix from me. Just be sure it has the protein powder in it.

George's Shake

2 cups milk, soy milk, or oat milk

½ cup fruit juice

2 tablespoons protein powder (choose a sugar-free one)

2 tablespoons oatmeal (not instant)

Put all ingredients in the blender and blend on high for about a minute. If you do it for less time, you will be crunching oats at the bottom of your shake. Using raw rolled oats is best. Don't use the steel-cut oats for this shake. If you prefer not to use milk of any sort in your shake, use 2 cups water and a little juice. George's Shake works because it combines nutritious foods with plenty of protein.

Whatever you choose to eat for breakfast, enjoy yourself! And make sure it has protein. Don't worry yet about making other changes like avoiding white-flour foods or taking the sugars out, just start with a regular breakfast that includes protein. We are working on creating a steady and stable blood sugar.

Ten Breakfast Ideas

Here are some other ideas for breakfast. Make a copy of this page, fold it up, and carry it with you in your wallet, appointment book, or purse. Flag this page so you can find it again.

1. Scrambled eggs and toast
2. Cottage cheese mixed with fresh fruit and a muffin
3. Pancakes or waffles made with protein powder in the batter
4. Two slices of toast with peanut butter
5. Cheese omelet with hash browns
6. Beef or chicken burrito
7. Oatmeal with milk or yogurt and fruit
8. Two hard-boiled eggs and juice to have in the car on the way to work

9. Bagel with lunch meat inside
10. Corned beef hash and two eggs with a slice of toast

Fast Food Breakfast Choices

For some of you, fast food places may be your only alternative. An Egg McMuffin is better than a doughnut and coffee. A Big Breakfast is even better. And yes, these are not ideal choices. But they will get you started and they will hold you until lunch. Because you are sugar sensitive, you are actually quite capable of finding what you need. You can remember times when you have gone out at 10 P.M. to find something sweet to eat because there was nothing in the house.

You can also find breakfasts in fast food restaurants. Actually, breakfast is one of the easiest meals to find on the road. Scrambled eggs and hash browns, an egg-and-cheese burrito, oatmeal (add your own protein powder that you carry in a Baggie), cottage cheese and fruit with some whole wheat toast. Go ahead and have the breakfast meat, too. You need a solid amount of protein.

Tips from the Field: The Power of Protein

I drink a George's Shake at breakfast, which gives me a big dose of protein. If I skip it, I crave sugars all day and eat and gain weight. I aim for the right amount of protein at every meal. If I'm consistent in that, and eating at regular intervals, my sugar cravings are minimal and I am *not hungry*.

—*L.*

A Shopping List to Cope with Chaos

Having the food you need to eat means actually having the food *in your house*. This means going to the grocery store and getting what you need. Planning and going grocery shopping regularly is the start of your making and carrying through conscious decisions about what you are going to eat. Right now it doesn't matter whether you put doughnuts and cookies in your cart as long as you are also buying breakfast foods and protein.

But start exercising your grocery-planning muscles. Your foggy and impulsive sugar-sensitive brain tends to take over when you are grocery shopping, causing you to come home with two boxes of breakfast streusel but without the carton of eggs you needed.

Before you go to the grocery store, write down what you are going to buy. This is the beginning of planning, a process you will get very good at. Start by sitting down and thinking about what you like to eat. This is important. Food meets your emotional as well as your physical needs. Enjoy the planning!

Once you have some notes on what you want to buy, make your shopping list match the layout of your grocery store. Choose the store you like to shop in. Sketch a picture of what your grocery store looks like. Add where the meats are, where the dairy counter is, where the fresh fruits and vegetables are. Then list the foods you want to buy in the order in which you pass them on your way through the store. This will keep you from being distracted and "drifting" toward sweet foods rather than consciously buying what you need for your plan.

When you first start this exercise, you may not know where the vegetables live. You may not have a good sense of your protein options. But mapping the layout will help you get the lay of the land in your own grocery store.

Tips to Help You Shop

Here are two more tips about grocery shopping:

- Don't shop when you're hungry.
- Don't shop when you're tired.

Try to go shopping *after* you've had a satisfying meal and at a time when you are not feeling exhausted or rushed. Now, if going to the grocery store is not the most exciting thing in the world for you, you will have to sort of will your way through this exercise. But it's easier if you are not tired and hungry when you go.

Even with the best-laid plans, however, sometimes you will be tired and hungry *and* need to buy groceries. Plan for this. Know what you will do. Maybe you will go back to the deli section and get something to eat before you start your main shopping. Maybe you will get a meal at a nearby restaurant, then hit the grocery store. If you eat first, you may still be tired but you will not be desperately hungry—and grabbing whatever sweet foods are at hand because of that hunger. You will make better choices and stick closer to your grocery list as you shop.

Your First Grocery List

You may not have a lot of experience with making a grocery list. You may be used to simply going to the store and picking out what calls to you. This time, try to think through the kinds of food you want to get before you go. If you need some help making a grocery list, start with this one. You may include other foods as well, but this is a core list.

A dozen eggs	Bread
Cottage cheese	A brick of cheese
Potatoes	Peanut butter
Triscuits	Apples or some other fruit

After you have gone grocery shopping several times you will be able to keep this list in your head. You will have the food you need on hand. Breakfast with protein will become a natural and habitual part of your daily routine. You can explore which of the breakfast choices you like most. Some people choose one breakfast and eat that every day. Others want to have something different every morning. Find what works best for you.

As you start to feel comfortable with your daily breakfast, begin to think about getting started with a food journal.

Step 2. Journal What You Eat and How You Feel

Your food journal is the cornerstone of your program. It may start out being a housekeeping task, but as you move through the program, it becomes a vital source of information about your body and your brain chemistry. Your journal is your body's voice.

Here are the basics of starting a food journal.

First, get yourself a blank book that you can carry with you. You might want to buy a diary with a zipper so you can feel safer about your privacy. The most important thing is to get something you feel comfortable with. Some folks use steno pads, some use fancy journals, some use their computers. Do whatever appeals to you most. While your computer may seem like an ideal alternative, writing your journal in longhand is better. The changes in your handwriting will give you clues about how you are doing with the program.

Write down in your journal what you eat or drink, when you eat or drink it, and how you feel physically and emotionally. Write down these feelings not only at the times you eat, but also whenever you notice them. For example, if you feel sleepy thirty minutes after lunch, write that down.

Use a four-column format for your food journal. Using four columns, you can easily see the connection between what you eat and how you feel physically and emotionally. Below is an example of a page of a food journal.

Date/ Time	What I Ate or Drank	How I Feel Physically	How I Feel Emotionally
April 10 8:00 A.M.	2 doughnuts	Tired	Really good
10:00 A.M.			Depressed. Feel like I can hardly function.
11:00 A.M.	2 cups of coffee with cream and sugar	Exhausted, can't stay awake	
1:00 P.M.			Really good
1:15 P.M.	Nachos Large Coke	Wired	Crabby about work
1:30 P.M.		Tense	
3:15 P.M.	2 cups of coffee with cream and sugar	Wired	Sad. How can I be sad and wired at the same time?
5:30 P.M.	2 beers	Relaxed, warm	Happy
7:00 P.M.	3 pieces of chicken, coleslaw, mashed potatoes, 2 biscuits with butter		Happy, satisfied, feel great

How the Simple Act of Writing Things Down Will Help

When you take the time to pay attention and make an entry in your food journal, you are giving energy to your own healing. You are telling your body it is important. You are noticing what you are eating and what you are feeling. You may think you don't need to write things down. You "know" what you eat. But when you actually start keeping a journal, you will be floored to discover that what you thought you knew and what you actually did were very different.

Keep the journal. It is an invaluable tool for understanding your own needs, rhythms, and changes.

Why Paying Attention Changes Things

When you pay attention to your body, you are sending it a message that it is valuable. If your body feels valuable, it will talk to you more. It will give you clearer messages and you can communicate better with each other. For too long, you have dismissed what your body feels. You have either ignored its signals or responded to its cues without being aware of what they really meant. There are likely many times you thought you were hungry when you were actually experiencing beta-endorphin withdrawal. Your journal will help you sort out what is really going on in your brain chemistry and your body.

What to Do If You Don't Know How You Feel

Some people have a hard time when they first start keeping their food journal because they honestly do not know how they feel. They get discouraged because all they are doing is writing "fine" or "okay" or sometimes "horrible" and "discouraged." This can happen because they have not listened to their bodies for so long. They have forgotten or never learned the language of feelings. Here is a list of the feelings you might experience.

Feeling Good

Able	Desirable	Playful
Alert	Determined	Pleasant
Challenged	Eager	Pleased
Animated	Enchanted	Powerful
Beautiful	Energetic	Proud
Bold	Energized	Radiant
Blissful	Excited	Real
Brave	Exhilarated	Refreshed
Brilliant	Free	Resilient
Bubbly	Full	Responsible
Buoyant	Fun	Responsive
Calm	Generous	Satisfied
Capable	Glad	Secure
Carefree	Grounded	Serene
Caring	Happy	Settled
Centered	Honored	Sexy
Cheerful	Humorous	Shining
Cherished	Impressed	Spiritual
Clean	Inspired	Spontaneous
Clear	Joyous	Thrilled
Clever	Loving	Stable
Confident	Open	Tenacious
Contented	Patient	Vital
Delighted	Peaceful	

Feeling Not So Good

Afraid	Burdened	Disappointed
Ambivalent	Cheated	Discontented
Angry	Childish	Disorganized
Annoyed	Combative	Distracted
Anxious	Confused	Distraught
Blue	Defeated	Disturbed
Bored	Destructive	Empty

Exasperated	Imposed upon	Restless
Exhausted	Inadequate	Sad
Explosive	Infuriated	Scared
Fearful	Jealous	Selfish
Flighty	Jumpy	Shocked
Foolish	Lonely	Shut down
Forgotten	Longing	Silent
Frantic	Mad	Skeptical
Frazzled	Miserable	Sleepy
Frightened	Nervous	Strange
Frustrated	Obsessed	Stupid
Grief-stricken	Outraged	Teary
Guilty	Overwhelmed	Tempted
Helpless	Panicked	Tense
High	Petrified	Terrible
Horrible	Pressured	Toxic
Hurt	Rejected	Unclear
Impatient	Resilient	Zonked

Go through this list and use a yellow highlighter to mark the feelings that seem to fit you best. You may find that there are only five to ten that fit where you are these days. Or you may highlight more than that if you know your feelings well. You may be discouraged because you really don't have feelings other than "fine" or "depressed." Keep reading the list as you keep your journal. Your ability to recognize feelings will change as your food changes.

The fun thing will be to see how your feelings emerge as you do the program. Whatever your feelings, the important thing is to notice—without criticizing yourself—that you are feeling something. Remember, words for feelings are not good or bad. They are simply a way to help you understand what is happening. You may be angry and frustrated at having to keep a food journal. Write this in your journal. You may be bored with your life. Write this in your journal. Your journal is your friend. It will teach you all about your wonderful body.

Remember that sugar-sensitive people tend to be people of extremes. You can feel either totally awash in feelings or totally disconnected. What you are trying to do is learn to notice and record. You do not have to sort it all out or make sense of the feelings. As you keep your journal, however, you might discover that there is a direct correlation between what you have been eating and how you are feeling.

Tips from the Field:
When the Body Speaks, Take Good Notes

Whenever I feel a strong emotion, I try to write it in the journal. Of course, some days it's one emotion after another, but generally I can identify specific strong emotions at various times throughout the day. I used to put "hungry" or "tired" a lot for the physical feelings that I recorded just before I ate. Then I realized I could use the physical and emotions columns any time—and, in fact, using those columns when it *wasn't* time to eat told me a lot more about myself and how food affected me. Writing in the journal at non-meal times helps me to listen to my body.

—L.

Learning to Read Your Body

Getting started with your journal will get you started with learning the language of your body. Begin to "listen" to the tones and new words of your body language. If you are not sure of the emotional content, focus on the physical. Try to notice when you are less tired or have more energy. If you usually have headaches and then notice you don't, make sure to write this down. If you usually have joint pains or rashes or a runny nose and notice that you're getting fewer of them, write this in your journal. If you simply use one word like "fine" to describe how you feel, it will be hard to sort out any change in your feelings.

Start by picking three feelings from the feelings list that you can comfortably relate to. Use them in your journal, then expand your list as you go. For example, I like to use the word "cranky" because it really conveys how I feel the next day if my food is off. It took me a while to find the right word to describe the feeling.

Doing It Every Day

Even if you hate doing the journal, do it anyway. Write down whatever you are feeling about the journaling process in the column labeled "How I feel emotionally." If you find you are still resisting doing a traditional journal, try a new approach. Use pictures, make a collage, draw images, use stickers. Experiment with alternatives that are less boring for you. Use a handheld recorder and then transcribe at the end of the day. Write in your appointment book. Be outrageous.

Tips from the Field: Making It Fun!

I use Crayola sparkly crayons (crayons that have glitter in them), as well as fluorescent gold stars, pink hearts, happy faces, etc., in my food journal. It's like doing a coloring book three times a day! Takes me back to being a child—and since I had such an awful childhood, I'm getting to do kid things now that I didn't get to do then. I know some folks on the program are actually drawing in their journals, but since I can't even draw a straight line, I rely on the neat stickers. In my emotional column I use pink or blue to reflect how I'm feeling. This really helps when I want to look back and see if there's a pattern.

—Y.

At some point, something will shift. All of a sudden instead of munching and writing and feeling mad, you will see the journal as your friend on the journey.

Managing the Intensity of Your Feelings

Sugar addicts often have volatile feelings. You may have been using sweet or white-flour-based foods to help you manage the chaos of your emotions. Your feelings may either be huge or nonexistent or swing back and forth between these two extremes. You may feel wild or numb. You may sometimes feel deeply and other times not at all. All of this is natural because of the imbalances in your brain and body chemistry. These feelings have been unmanageable because they have come without warning or pattern. This is going to change. You will discover that there are very predictable patterns as to why and when you feel the way you do. What has seemed like chaos will change into fascinating connections between your food and your mood.

It is natural for you to be scared or to want to rush ahead. You are not alone. All sugar addicts feel this way. Much of what you feel is shaped by how you have been eating. When your meals are erratic, when you are eating lots of white-flour foods and are still having a sugar life, sugar feelings—feelings of chaos and doom—will emerge. Seeing impediments rather than solutions; feeling many fears and doubts; wanting to start, being terrified of starting; being impatient, being resistant; being wildly enthusiastic—all these feelings will surface. All the feelings are real, but they are amplified by the unbalanced biochemistry. These are not bad feelings, they are sugar feelings. Be kind as you learn to identify them.

The good news is the sugar feelings will change. Your feelings will still be deep, but they will no longer scare you. They will be manageable and understandable. They will work in your service rather than making you crazy. This is one of the most exciting benefits of sticking with your plan and "doing the food."

You will be able to simply work the steps of the plan before you understand everything. You will learn to listen to your body and live without knowing the rationale for each recommendation while you are sorting things out. It will get better over time. What has been scary will become safe, and you will understand what you feel.

4

Getting Steady:
Steps 3 and 4

This phase of your program is designed to help you get stable.
It is about adding new foods and new ideas, paying attention, and getting into a rhythm. Don't even be thinking about what you are *not* going to be able to eat, because you will not be giving anything up until you and your body are ready. Your body will guide you as we go through the steps. First, you want to stabilize your sugar-sensitive body chemistry.

Stability requires building a firm foundation before starting to build new structures on top of it. Now that you feel you have found a solution to your symptoms, you probably want to get on with the whole program all at once. You want to get rid of the sugar right now. Hold that enthusiasm in check and keep reading.

You may vacillate between wanting to give up all your sugar this moment and being terrified at the thought of never eating sugar again. This is natural and to be expected. Move away from thinking that *sugar* is creating the mood swings, depression, and addiction. Your unbalanced biochemistry sets you up, and what you eat makes it worse. The problem is much bigger than just the sugar itself. In this phase, we want to stabilize both your body and your behavior. We are going to slow you down and simply begin to retrain some of your old patterns. We will harness your impulsivity, minimizing the urge to make huge changes all at once, while still preserving your delightful spontaneity. Slow and thoughtful will be our theme for this task.

Step 3. Eat Three Meals a Day with Protein

I am a patient woman who has worked with thousands and thousands of sugar-sensitive people. On the Sugar Addict's Total Recovery Program, every client takes small steps so that the plan works. I want you to go slow enough, too, that you can master each little change. I know that every one of these changes will have a dramatic impact on how you feel. They are the foundation for lifelong change.

Hopefully, you now are eating breakfast with protein every morning, ideally within one hour of waking up. This may have been a huge step for you. Sometimes it takes weeks to master this simple beginning because it is so easy to skip breakfast. Having the protein with your breakfast makes a huge difference in how you feel. If you have been able to get started in this way, I suspect you are beginning to feel a bit better already.

The next step is to eat three meals a day with protein, at about the same time every day, such as 7:30 A.M., 12:30 P.M., and 5:30 P.M. Or 7:00 A.M., noon and 6:00 P.M. Try to have no more than five to six hours between each meal (except for the overnight stretch between dinner and breakfast). If you are going to have to go longer than that, consider having a protein and complex carbohydrate snack to tide you over. For example, if you suspect you will have to work late and not be able to get dinner until 8:00 P.M., think about this in the afternoon or whenever this suspicion first arises. Plan to get a snack of protein and complex carbs by 5:00 P.M. You want to make sure to keep your body from crashing in a big way. (This is the exception to my usual advice of not eating between meals.)

A normal person would just get hungry. A normal person would say at 5:30, "I'm starving. I have to get something to eat." But our bodies respond to blood sugar depletion in a different way. Our bodies cue into the serious blood sugar drop and say, "Whoa, starvation may be coming. I gotta protect this loved one." And our body releases beta-endorphin so we'll feel better. We end up feeling emotionally wonderful, euphoric, relaxed, thin, and self-confident by *not* eating when we need to.

You may mistakenly think that this "good" feeling is something to strive for. But the "good" feeling comes as your body acts to protect you from what it thinks is happening. It thinks you are starving and doesn't want you to suffer. It releases a painkiller: our friend beta-endorphin. You know how much you love beta-endorphin! However, not eating as a way to get a beta-endorphin high is a dangerous tactic. It can set you up for anorexic patterns. This is *not* the direction we want your healing to take.

Because of this particular beta-endorphin response, when you first give up your pattern of not eating, you may experience beta-endorphin withdrawal and edginess. Don't get spooked, just understand what is happening.

The wonderful beta-endorphin feeling of being able to go forever without eating masks trouble in another way as well. You may continue to push yourself until your beta-endorphin supply runs low. Your blood sugar continues to drop. Then you suddenly realize you are in big trouble. Now the warmth of the beta-endorphin is gone *and* the pain of the blood sugar drop hits. You eat anything—sometimes everything in sight. And if you're in the early months of this plan, "anything in sight" may well be white, sweet, and trouble.

Often people say to me, "But I don't get hungry. Why should

I eat if I am not hungry?" Sugar-sensitive people don't always register hunger the way normal people do. Your hunger thermostat may not be working properly. If it isn't, you may not feel hunger, and you may not feel full after eating. This will change over time, but in the early stages of this program, you will need to serve as your own clock by eating at regularly scheduled intervals. You have to compensate for your own low level of serotonin. You will need to pay close attention to the time. Use your journal to help you start to notice when you are likely to get into trouble from going too long between meals.

If for some reason you get a meal off your regular time, simply shift back to your routine. Don't confuse your body. Reinforce the *pattern* of your eating. For example, if you couldn't get lunch until 2:00 P.M., still have your dinner at the regular time. Remember, consistency and regularity is what we are striving for. We are looking to get those meals into regular slots, not at random intervals.

This part of your program will be hard. Sometimes it takes people months to really master it. Consistency and stability are somewhat alien to the typical sugar sensitive. We often put our own needs last. This characteristic seems to be a part of sugar sensitivity. This may make us good caretakers, but it leaves that wonderful body of ours pretty low on the list. I encourage people to think of their body as a three-year-old child's body. You wouldn't make a three-year-old skip a meal or wait too long to eat. You would stop what you were doing and make dinner for the little one. *Do this for yourself.*

Create regular mealtimes. Remember, regular mealtimes.

Regular Protein Is Crucial

Each of your three meals needs to contain a good amount of protein. This plan is *not* a high-protein plan; it is a regular and consistent protein plan. Having protein consistently throughout the day does two key things: It helps to stabilize your blood sugar because protein is a very "slow" food, and it creates a steady state of amino acids in your body.

Most sugar-sensitive people on the program are eating about 5 ounces of a protein (like beef, fish, or chicken) at each meal. If you want to count protein grams, aim for 0.4 to 0.6 grams of protein for each pound of your weight for your total daily allotment. An easy way to figure this out is to take half your body weight as your daily "gram" allotment. Divide that by 3 to get a sense of how many grams of protein to eat at each meal. For example, if you weigh 150 pounds, you will have a total of 75 grams of protein each day, or 25 grams per meal. If you decide to count grams of protein, you will need to get a book, table, or nutrition software to tell you the grams of protein in the foods you typically eat.

If you are a counter, be careful not to get into trouble spending all your time trying to figure out exactly what to eat rather than enjoying the eating. You may get confused in trying to convert grams to ounces. Protein foods are usually sold or prepared as ounce servings. The food contains things like water and fat, so it is hard to sort out the exact amount of grams of protein in a given food.

I encourage people to start simply by using an easy "eyeball" method. Simply make a fist. That is about how much protein you want to have at a meal. Two eggs, a good-sized piece of fish, a good-sized breast of chicken. (This is more than the traditional "pack of cards" portion size used in some weight-loss programs.) If you have a bigger fist, you will eat more; if you have a smaller fist, you will eat less.

We are working really hard to shift your awareness about food. I want you to think about what you are eating rather than simply wolfing down your food unconsciously. I want you to be thinking about the enjoyment of the chicken breast rather than whether it is 4.5 ounces or 5.7 ounces. We sugar sensitives sometimes get stuck on little things and forget about the why of eating.

Do not count anything but protein foods as your protein. For example, don't count the amount of protein in bread or breakfast cereal as part of your daily protein. Even though they contain some protein, bread and breakfast cereal are carbohydrates, not proteins. Don't think of milk as protein either. Yes, I know it has protein in it. But it is pretty light on the protein scale and won't really hold you for very long.

A good way to start with making sure you get enough protein is to make a list for yourself of the foods you like and generally eat as your protein foods. Protein foods include things like eggs, dairy products, cottage cheese, peanut butter, lentils, tofu, beef, lamb, chicken, and fish. (If you are vegetarian, you can surely do the plan, but you will need to pay close attention to what you are eating to make sure you get enough protein.)

Figure out the portion size for those foods to get the grams of protein you need per meal, then use that list for planning your meals. For example, my list contains things like this:

- Two eggs
- 5-ounce turkey burger
- 5 ounces of salmon fillet
- 7 ounces of cottage cheese
- 8 ounces of tofu (soy is less dense as a protein than animal foods)
- One medium chicken breast
- 5 ounces of ground beef in spaghetti sauce
- 6 ounces of tuna salad (one can of tuna)
- Two veggie burgers (I never looked at the box to read the protein count—it just feels right)
- A 1-inch slice of meatloaf
- 12 ounces of a protein shake (24 grams of protein provided by 2 tablespoons of protein powder)

Now, how do I figure out what 7 ounces of cottage cheese looks like, or 5 ounces of ground turkey? I buy the turkey in half-pound (8-ounce) packages and eat a little more than half the package at a meal. I know that cottage cheese comes in 8-ounce tubs, so I leave some and I put it on my dog's dinner. I read the size of the original salmon fillet and cut off what looks like 5 ounces. By now you may have guessed I am not a counter-type person. But I have found what works for me. Your job is to sort out what works *for you.* We want it to be fun and easy.

Protein is key for your body to repair itself. Also remember that protein provides your body with tryptophan, the amino acid that your body needs to make serotonin. If you aren't eating protein, your serotonin factory will have to go on layoff status.

Tips from the Field: Making Protein Easy

For protein, I use chicken breasts, turkey breasts, steak, eggs, and bacon and ground beef. When I get home from the store, I separate the breasts into individual plastic bags and freeze them, so I can grab one at a time if I need to.

When I cook them, I usually cook about four servings at a time, eat one and keep the other three in the fridge or freezer.

I've used ground beef for meatloaf and cabbage rolls that I make without the added sugars and white flour, instead adding more veggies. I always try to make extras so that I have something for lunch or breakfast or for those dinners when the whole family is off on their own activities.

—M.

So pay attention to the protein at your meals. And remember, we are not talking about high-protein meals here. We are talking about regular and consistent meals centered on protein. The meal needs to contain other things as well as the protein. A balance of protein, complex carbohydrates, and fats is important. But at this stage, we are only working on getting protein into each of your three meals a day.

What Is a Meal?

Let's take a look at what you will be eating with your protein. What is a meal? A "meal" is eating two or more nutritious foods at one sitting. At a minimum, a meal should consist of a complex carbohydrate and a protein. Here are some meals:

- Tuna fish and salad with vegetables (lettuce alone is kind of light)
- Eggs and toast or an Egg McMuffin with hash browns
- Chicken breast and green beans
- Three tacos
- Hamburger and corn
- Cottage cheese and tomatoes
- Chili on brown rice
- A bean-and-cheese burrito
- Fish cakes and a baked potato
- Lentil soup and a baked potato
- Beef stew with carrots and peas in it
- A bagel with lox and cream cheese
- Club sandwich, celery sticks, potato chips
- A protein shake made with milk, fruit, and protein powders based on vegetable, soy, egg, or whey or a combination

Now, you may be shocked at some of the "meals" I have listed. Remember, I told you that I am patient. I want you to succeed on this plan. I want you to start where you are, not where I or anyone else thinks you should be. Start with your lifestyle. As you feel better, you will begin to want to make more informed meal choices. Besides, if you start to feel like I am taking away everything you love to eat, you will either resent me or not do the program (or both). What I want is for you to start with what you can do.

Have Sweets with Your Meal and Don't Worry About It

As we are starting to talk about meals, you are probably wondering when you have to give up the sugar stuff. You know it's coming sometime and you are no doubt giving that fear a lot of energy. You may be going back and forth between being raring to go and dumping it all and being terrified that I am going to take away your support. Actually, at this stage, we will do neither.

At this point in the program, don't even think about giving up your friends, the sugar foods. For now, simply eat your sweets as part of your meals. If you usually eat a candy bar in the afternoon, just eat it earlier with lunch or later with your dinner. If you have an almond croissant for breakfast, just have it with a breakfast that contains protein (such as eggs) and a complex carbohydrate (such as whole wheat toast). The other foods in your meal will slow down the effect of the candy or sweet foods. You will have less of a hit or rush from the sugars you eat with meals, but you can keep your friends at your side for now. Remember, though, they are now an add-on, not part of your meal. I once had someone ask me if a hot fudge sundae counted as a meal since it was two or more nutritious foods and included foods with protein in it (ice cream and nuts). She was serious. Only a sugar-sensitive person would think this way. We are so creative in finding a way to keep our beloved foods. The answer is, a sundae isn't a meal.

Tips from the Field: If You're Overdue for a Meal

If I find myself getting past due on a meal and I just can't (for any reason) get it together to make myself a meal, I either eat what I can get
(a hard-boiled egg, a hunk of cheese, cottage cheese, maybe a piece
of fruit—usually fruit and cheese or nuts are best to perk me up
when I am crashing) or drop everything and go to a restaurant.

—D.

Why Only Three Meals? And Why No Snacks?

What's wrong with having a snack? Like cheese and Triscuits in
the late afternoon, or half a protein shake mid-morning? Some
people have even been encouraged to maintain an even blood
sugar level by having six small meals a day rather than three big
ones. Why do I say to eat three times a day?

You and I have a special sugar-sensitive body chemistry. Saying no is not our strongest suit. It is very easy for us to go from
having "just a little snack" to grazing throughout the day. We
start eating and forget to stop. I am teaching your body how to
start and stop. When you end a meal and consciously *stop eating*,
you are helping your dear, sweet addictive body to learn something new and good. Stopping is healthy.

For most of us, having no control—not being able to say no
and being impulsive—is a problem. We have huge pain and
shame around it. It is behavior we want to change. I have found
that if we make simple choices and quiet the old negative messages we have about what we should or should not be doing, we
can change old patterns. Three meals (starting and stopping)
seem to do this really well.

Of course, there are a few exceptions to the recommendation of only three meals. As you follow this plan, you will start to

see that we are not working with rules so much as guidelines. I want you to be thinking about what is right for you. I want you to understand *why* I recommend certain changes.

However, if you are pregnant or nursing or engaging in major athletic activity or you are a growing teen, you will *need* to snack. And if you have to go more than six hours without a meal, have a planned snack.

Choose snacks that combine protein and a complex carbohydrate. Here are some sample snacks:

- A hard-boiled egg and a cut-up orange
- Mozzarella sticks with corn chips and salsa
- Triscuits (or some other whole grain cracker) and bean dip
- An ounce of cheddar cheese and an apple
- A slice of whole grain toast with peanut butter
- String cheese and spicy V-8 juice

Don't fret a lot about this; just choose the best snacks for your lifestyle.

What About Diet Soda, Tea, or Coffee Between Meals?

As you start to work with the idea of three meals a day, you will wonder about what to drink between meals. Just start to pay attention to the between-meal time. You want to be careful not to drift toward substituting coffee or soda for the foods you used to eat during the day.

You also want to pay attention to your social times. So much of our social culture revolves around having something to drink together; it may seem hard to imagine life without it. At this stage in your program, don't stop drinking anything. Don't even think of giving everything up today. Do not spook yourself.

Just start noticing your pattern—what you drink and when you drink it. Notice the triggers and the amounts. Write about the drinks in your journal.

Grocery Shopping

In order to manage having three meals a day with protein, you will need to go grocery shopping. When we live in sugar chaos, we often just eat what is in the house, or we grab something on the way home, or we go grocery shopping when we have already missed a meal and are "off the cliff."

All of these conditions contribute to chaos and will not support stability and consistency in your plan. I want you to begin to learn to plan what meals you are going to eat. I am going to show you how to prepare a shopping list so you have what you need to make those meals, and then actually go into a grocery store when you are neither tired nor hungry and purchase what you need. You are smiling, aren't you? You *know* this will be a radical change from your usual grocery behavior.

Getting Ready to Go Grocery Shopping

Let's start with planning. Think about three meals a day for the time period you will be shopping for. Do you shop once a week, every day, or once a month? Whatever suits your pattern, sit down and think through what you will need for those three meals a day. If you don't have a shopping pattern at all, I suggest you plan to shop once a week. Plan to get the basic food you need. You may go out for a meal during the week or you may stop quickly at the market to add to what you've already bought, but doing your main grocery shopping once a week will give you the basic foods you need to stay safe with your food plan.

Sit down and make a little chart for yourself. Make seven columns and then draw two horizontal lines across them. This will give you twenty-one spaces—three meals a day for one week. Fill in what kinds of things you think you might eat at each time of each day. This is *not* a food plan. It is simply a realistic assessment of your week. If you eat lunch from the truck that stops near your office every day, that's fine. Write in "truck lunch," and you will know you don't have to shop for those meals. If you usually go for a latte and something in the morning, just figure on whether the something includes enough protein. You may just be adding a hard-boiled egg. Then you will add eggs to your shopping list.

This is neither rocket science nor the thirty-day *Family Circle* meal plan. It's a quick sketch to help you figure out what to buy. After you have filled in the boxes, look at your chart. Start writing down the ingredients for the foods that you have filled in. This may include oatmeal, hamburger, soup, bread, and brownies (remember, you can have your sweet stuff—you are just going to be eating it *with* your meals). Then go see if you already have any of the things on your list. If you have plenty of oatmeal, you don't need to buy more.

You may find you would like to begin experimenting with things that are a little healthier than what you have been eating. If you want to do this, it's great, but you don't have to.

Make sure your list includes emergency food. I always get cottage cheese, for example, even though I may not have it on my eating list. If I get home late one night and feel run over by a truck (usually because it's way beyond mealtime), I can fix a baked potato in the microwave, add some cottage cheese, and slice a tomato for dinner. Other emergency foods for when there is no time to cook are canned tuna, Triscuits (or other whole wheat or rye crackers) with tuna and veggies, cheese sticks and veggies, natural peanut butter on a whole wheat tortilla or bread, or bagged salad with lunch meat and cheese.

Not ideal, but functional. If you have a potato for dinner, it doesn't count as your evening spud. If you eat late, you may want to cut your dinner potato in half and save half for the evening spud. Remember, the evening one before bed should have no protein foods with it.

A Sample Grocery List

So let's look at what you might have on your shopping list.

Proteins

Tuna I always keep several cans of tuna in my cupboard.

Chicken I usually get a combination of regular chicken breasts to bake and some boneless, skinless cutlets to use for a stir-fry or something. I usually get a whole chicken to roast on Sunday. Takes me back to my early days as a young wife. And makes the kitchen smell good.

Ground meat (I get either turkey or beef) I have them package it in the weight that is the right amount for a meal. Then I can stick them in the freezer and know I am prepared. Having it ground makes it easy to use for different things: in spaghetti sauce, on the grill, in meatloaf, etc.

Fish I generally get several different kinds of fish and put it in the freezer. Before I freeze it, I package it in individual serving sizes and label it.

Eggs I always have eggs in the refrigerator.

Cottage cheese This is another staple for me.

Tofu Again, I always keep some around because it is so easy and quick to fix.

Dairy things such as **cheese** and **plain yogurt** can be very helpful for your plan. They provide comfort and nourishment. Get **milk** if you drink it. It can be a good base for protein shakes if you decide to use them. Choose regular cow's milk or soy milk or oat milk. Stay away from rice milk, because it tends to be very sweet and may trigger cravings.

Vegetables

Ah, vegetables. I know that many sugar-sensitive people don't exactly thrive on veggies. But there are a few that you can start with no matter what.

Get at Store

Tuna: 2 big cans	Spinach
Chicken breasts	Lettuce
Roaster chicken	Lentil soup
Hamburger: 2 pounds	Bread
Salmon	Oatmeal
A dozen eggs	Potatoes
Cottage cheese	Carrots
Butter	Coffee beans

Potatoes   Make sure you have enough for your evening spud. Have fun with potatoes. Try different kinds; choose different colors and shapes. You are going to start noticing different tastes in potatoes. Yukon golds are very different from Idaho russets. Some folks swear that organic baking potatoes taste best. Become a potato connoisseur.

Go to the frozen food section. See which vegetables seem okay to you. **Peas** and **corn** are fine. You don't have to eat brussels sprouts. (The frozen ones are pretty bad.) Don't make yourself cranky about this. Don't go faster than you can go. If the only vegetables you eat are peas and corn, that's okay.

After you are finished in the frozen food section, wander down to the fresh vegetable section. Get a bag of **lettuce**. Get a little bag if you live alone; we want to minimize things turning brown and wilted (and becoming unappealing!) in the back of your refrigerator. Consider a salad. Maybe just lettuce, **tomato**, and **carrots**. Think about what you might like. See which vegetables call to you. They may be thrilled to meet you. They may clamor to hop into your cart and go home with you.

Fruits

After you have looked at the veggies, move over to the fruit section. We know the fruits will sing to you: **oranges, apples, bananas, peaches**. Choose the ones you like. Try different kinds and colors. Don't even think about whether the fruit is right for your plan. Just get what appeals to you. If you don't know how to pick out ripe fruit, ask the person in charge of produce.

Staples

Now you are going to walk around and get the staples that are important for your own plan. This may include **oatmeal**, **soup**, and **frozen entrées**. Use your list to guide you. Look around the supermarket and find food you are drawn to and will eat. Do *not* choose based on what you think is good for you. Choose what you like and will eat.

I had one client who could not master breakfast. He did this exercise and found something called cha-cha chili in those cardboard cups you add hot water to. He started having cha-cha chili for breakfast and felt 100 percent better. So look for things that are fun that you may not have noticed before. For example, if you get tortillas, you can make all sorts of meals wrapped in a tortilla. If you are choosing cereals, begin to hunt out the ones that are a little lower in sugar. Shredded Wheat and Cheerios will hold you better through the morning than Count Chocula. Oatmeal is the best.

Identifying Your Own Lifesavers

Identify a few lifesavers for yourself. (No, I don't mean the candy.) Pick out a few things that you will always have on hand in case you get into trouble with your food. For example, I always have **potatoes, oatmeal, cottage cheese, eggs**, and **rice cakes** at home. So even if I am not diligent, or I forget to get to the store and it's the sixth day and I am tired and cranky, I can make a meal of scrambled eggs and rice cakes. Everyone will have different lifesavers. But identify yours and get them at the store. And pay attention. If you use them up, make sure to get more! Your food lifesavers are as important as keeping extra toilet paper in the house. (Put that on your grocery list as well!)

Avoiding Fuzzy Foods

When you are shopping, think carefully about what you are getting. We want to avoid fuzzy food syndrome. If you find that some food you thought was going to be a big hit ends up in a plastic container in the back of your refrigerator with fur on it, don't keep using this food.

For example, I love the look and feel of eggplant. I used to buy an eggplant every week. And every week it would get spotted and soft, then mushy, and I would throw it out. I did this for many months until I figured out that I love to eat eggplant but hate to cook it. Now I get eggplant at a Chinese restaurant. Well, sometimes I bring the leftovers home and *they* get furry, but I am sure you understand what I mean. The bottom line? Stop the fuzzies. If it has been there for three days, throw it out.

Step 4. Eat a Potato Before Bed

Okay, let's assume you are now eating breakfast with protein every day. You may also have started to get to the grocery store regularly. You may even be doing some planning. This is a terrific beginning. Let's add Mr. Spud to your routine.

Have a potato (with its skin) every night just before bed. This may sound simple, but it will help your body raise your serotonin level and make you feel more confident, competent, creative, and optimistic. Big results from a single nightly spud, huh?

You can eat your potato baked, mashed, roasted, cut into oven fries, or grated into hash browns. Just be sure you eat the skin. And you can top it with anything you like *except* foods that contain a protein. (Protein eaten along with the potato at bedtime will interfere with your serotonin-making process.) Good toppings are butter, margarine, salsa, mustard, spices, olive oil, or flaxseed oil. Toppings you should *not* use are cheese, sour cream, bacon bits, or cream of chicken soup.

Your nightly spud does not have to be a big potato. It can be a russet, a Russian fingerling, or a little red potato. Experiment. I use a medium Yukon Gold with its skin on. If you find that you are having wild dreams on the nights you have your potato, this is a clue that you have low serotonin. This means you are getting a bigger hit of serotonin than you want right yet. The bigger hit means your levels are very low. You need the serotonin, but it is better to go more slowly. Ease into it and let your brain catch up. Have a smaller potato, or eat just a half or even a third of it. Your body is talking to you. Listen.

You may believe that a potato has a high glycemic index and will make you fat if you eat it before bed. Poor Mr. Spud has been given some bad press in the past few years. Recent books that suggest you use the glycemic index as a way to decide what to eat tell you potatoes raise your blood sugar very high. Potatoes are not bad, however.

Mashed potatoes *without* skin do have a very high glycemic index. Baked potatoes *with* the skin have a lower glycemic index but still have a glycemic punch. This is exactly why baked potatoes are perfect for the job. They evoke a glycemic response that causes a release of insulin to get that tryptophan into your brain to make serotonin. If you choose a carbohydrate that is too slow (that is to say, one with a very low GI), you will not get the desired effect. We will talk about potatoes and why they work more in Chapter 5, where I answer virtually every potato question you might have ever thought of.

When you get further along in the program, you'll find out

all sorts of options and choices about making your nightly potato more exciting. For now, just keep it simple. Eat a potato and its skin before bed.

Tips from the Field: Potato Particulars

I have found that a small spud is all it takes. You can bake it, pan-fry it, oven-fry it, or make potato salad from it. You can use leftover skin-on mashed spuds and make potato pancakes if you wish. Yes, you must eat the skin and you may use butter or oil on it—just no protein like cheese or sour cream.

—S.

Take Three Vitamins

Vitamins play an important role in helping your body through the sugar detox phase, and we'll talk a lot more about them later. For now, as part of Step 4, take these three:

1. Vitamin C: 500 to 5,000 mg a day (depending upon what you are used to)
2. Vitamin B complex: Choose one that is a 50-mg-a-day dosage. You might want to use a liquid formula because you can split the dose if you need to. Don't take it on an empty stomach or in the evening. If you feel a little buzzed by it, take less.
3. Zinc: 15 mg a day. Make sure to take your zinc with food. It can make you feel sick to your stomach if it is taken on an empty stomach. (Sucking on a zinc lozenge helps slow down and ease cold symptoms. If you are getting sick, you can increase the dose to 30 mg a day.)

If you're already taking a daily multivitamin, read the label and see if it contains the vitamin levels listed above. If so, simply keep taking it every day without any added supplements. If not, you may want to buy additional vitamins to make sure you are getting this baseline.

Many people ask me about taking more supplements, herbs, amino acids, or other minerals in addition to those in the plan. If you have identified a need for many of these things in developing a well-balanced and healthy life for yourself, you need not stop taking them. However, often people who are addicted are very fond of taking something rather than eating meals and making life changes. To change these behavior patterns, I encourage you to "do the food" as your first and primary commitment. After you have mastered the seven steps, then you can explore additions to your plan.

5

Getting the Details Sorted Out: Answers to Your Questions

Usually when people are starting out on their food plan, they have all sorts of questions for me. The sugar-sensitive brain is generally smart and curious. When it comes to food, it is even smarter and more curious. In addition, most people who follow this plan have read many books on diets and nutrition before finding this one. They may have lots of questions about how sugar sensitivity and diets work.

That's why I am devoting this chapter to answering the questions I hear most frequently. Some of the questions (and answers) may not be relevant for you yet, but they will iron out ahead of time some of the wrinkles you will probably be faced with as you progress through the program.

Is This a High-Fat Diet?

No. It is a moderate, healthy-fat plan. Your body needs fat for some of its most essential functions. The kind of fat you use has a huge impact on your health. Increase the good fats like olive oil, flaxseed oil, and fish oils, and reduce saturated fats found in foods such as meats and cheese. If you have been focusing on low-fat for a while and counting fat grams, this will be a change. That's because low-fat generally means high-sugar. I am trying to take the sugars out and increase the fat a little by steering you to the healthy ones.

Some people do find themselves eating more fat when they start the program. Fat, like sugar, is linked to the beta-endorphin system. Sugar-sensitive people may well have a beta-endorphin release in response to eating fat: they feel confident, competent, and optimistic after they have a meal higher in fat. This can be a good thing. Raising your beta-endorphin without getting a blood sugar spike (and its resulting steep drop) can help tide you over.

However, if you find yourself dreaming about high-fat foods, you will need to be careful that you don't transfer your beta-endorphin interest from sugar to fat. If your meals start drifting to nuts and cheese and more nuts and cheese, you know fat is calling you.

Isn't This Too Much Protein?

No. This is *not* a high-protein plan. It is a regular and consistent protein plan. The amount of protein I recommend is only a bit higher than the USDA recommended daily allowance (RDA). The RDA calls for 54 grams of protein a day for a 150-lb person, or a little less than 0.4 grams per pound of body weight. I recommend that sugar-sensitive people on my program have between 0.4 and 0.6 grams per pound of body weight, depending on their health needs. In the early stages of your recovery, your body may have more repair work to do and you may need to eat more protein. You would be eating at the upper end of what I recommend. Later, as you feel better, you can reduce the amount.

But overall, I try to move people away from counting, whether it's grams of fat or grams of protein. Counting has played such havoc with our bodies. Counting has been the center of most diets. I would prefer that you use the size of your fist to guide you in determining how much protein to eat at each meal. (It works like this: Hold out your hand and make a fist. Look at its size. Then eat a fist-sized portion of protein at each meal. Obviously, if you weigh more or have a bigger fist, you will need to eat more protein.)

Why Don't You Call This Plan "*Protein* Not Prozac"?

The protein is essential, but so is the potato. This is a *two-part* biochemical healing process: first the protein, then the potato. The protein gets tryptophan into your bloodstream. The potato before bed gets that tryptophan across the blood-brain barrier and into your brain, where your serotonin factory is located. More tryptophan means more serotonin, which will increase your optimism, your creativity, and your ability to concentrate. (If you want more details, read the next question.)

Questions on How Eating the Potato Works

What is the potato doing for my neurochemistry?

The potato is simply creating an insulin response, which has an effect on the movement of the amino acid tryptophan from your blood into your brain.

Why do we care about that? Because your body uses tryptophan to make serotonin. Serotonin is the brain chemical that makes you feel mellow and happy. It also helps you to "just say no" to sweets and other things by putting the brakes on your impulsivity.

Tryptophan is a kind of amino acid that comes from protein. When you eat protein foods (meats, cheese, eggs, poultry, etc.), they are broken down into amino acids. These amino acids go into your bloodstream and try to get into the brain as brain food. One of these aminos, tryptophan, is a little runt. The other amino acids, the big ones, compete with him and won't let him get across into the brain.

But there's an exception. When you eat a food (like a potato) that causes an insulin reaction, the insulin grabs the big amino acids and carries them off to your muscles as muscle food. The muscles don't really care about the runt, tryptophan, so he gets left behind in the bloodstream. Without the competition of the big aminos, little tryptophan can hop across the blood-brain barrier into the brain, where it will be used to produce serotonin. Thus, your serotonin levels rise.

So I want you to eat protein with dinner, then three hours later have something to raise your insulin level. A potato seems like a better alternative than a candy bar.

If you eat a bigger potato, will you get more serotonin?

Lots of people ask this. Then they take it a step further and ask, "If you eat lots of protein *and* the big potato, will you get even more serotonin? Is there a limit to this? If one is good, two must be better!"

If you have had good protein at dinner three hours earlier, it is likely that a big potato will stoke the serotonin factory more. However, seeking a bigger hit is not the aim of the potato task. Bigger protein amounts and larger potatoes are not the goal. A hit of serotonin that is too much may cause you nightmares and give you a hangover. This is definitely not a "more is better" thing. You're just after a good night's sleep and a gentle rise in your overall serotonin level.

If you are already taking an antidepressant, you may find that you do not need to use a large potato. In fact, if you do, you may increase the side effects of your antidepressant. Your sleep may become restless, you may have a headache, or you may find you are less able to have an orgasm. You have two options: decrease the size of the potato or talk with your doctor about decreasing the amount of antidepressant you are taking. If you decide to do this, do it slowly and carefully.

If I don't notice any differences in my mood, should I eat a bigger potato the next night?

Play around a bit and see what happens. The effects from food usually aren't as dramatic as the effects from drugs. They are often more subtle and build over time. But most sugar-sensitive people love to experiment. It's harmless with the potato.

Why do I have weird dreams since I started eating the potato?

The potato is increasing your serotonin level, which is related to REM sleep and dreaming. These changes in your dreams mean the spud is working! This should change in a week or so. If the dreams disturb you, use a smaller potato.

The potato seems to give me a headache. Why?

You might need to decrease the amount of potato you are eating. Too much serotonin can cause a headache. This may be a clue that your "dose" is not right.

Are there any other ways I can increase serotonin by using food and/or timing?

Once you understand the principles of the protein/carbohydrate timing, you can work out a plan that best suits you. Master the basics of having regular, consistent protein and a timed carbohydrate.

If I want to get more serotonin in the winter (I have SAD—seasonal affective disorder), should I eat a potato three hours after lunch and after dinner?

For people who are severely depressed, I will sometimes recommend that they actually have a second (or even a third) carbohydrate snack (three hours after each meal). This is simply to maximize the serotonin effect. Experiment to see if it helps. You don't need to eat a lot of potato, but do pay attention to *when* you eat it.

Will the potato let me stop taking my antidepressants?

The potato helps raise your serotonin levels. Some people have found that doing the food plan (not just the potato at night) has a huge impact on how they feel. They ask me whether they should just stop taking their medication. My recommendation is to do the food plan for at least six months. If you feel you are ready to reduce or stop your medication, talk with your doctor to plan a gradual taper. Some people are able to go off their medication with the food plan. Others are able to reduce their dosage. And others keep taking their medication but find it works more effectively. Your job is to understand the biochemistry of your body and your needs and then use the food plan and medications to get the result you want.

Is the potato considered one of my three meals?

No. The first phase of the program is to eat three meals a day with protein, *plus* a potato before bed. The potato is not a snack so much as a medicinal intervention.

Can I eat potatoes with meals as well?

Of course. Just be sure to eat the skin.

What should I do if I miss the potato?

If you mean for one night, don't worry about it. If you start forgetting a lot, figure out what you can do to remind yourself. It is an important part of the plan.

Does it have to be a potato?

Well, yes and no. The potato is ideal. This is why I called my first book *Potatoes Not Prozac*, rather than *Triscuits Not Prozac* or *Apples Not Prozac*. Also, potatoes are a very good comfort food. Think of the spud as number one. If you simply can't do the spud (some people are allergic to them), here are some good alternatives:

- Baked sweet potatoes with butter, cinnamon, and nutmeg (without skin)
- Triscuits with butter
- Brown rice with butter, cinnamon, and nutmeg
- Oatmeal
- Oven-fried sweet spuds (without the skin)
- Skin-on sugar-free potato salad
- Brown rice cakes with some butter

Remember, as with the spud, don't have any protein with these nighttime carbohydrates.

What if I'm diabetic?

If you are diabetic, don't use the white potato; use a sweet potato or one of the alternatives above.

Don't potatoes have a high glycemic index? Won't they spike my blood sugar?

Yes, potatoes do evoke insulin, although when they are eaten with their skins, they raise the blood sugar far more slowly than what is reported as the glycemic index, which was developed with mashed potatoes (without skins and without butter). But remember, we *want* a timed insulin response to get that trypto-phan from your blood into your brain!

You really do not have to worry about the glycemic index of one potato. Going off all the sweet foods you have been eating will create a hefty impact on your health.

The skin protects you further. It is mostly fiber and dramati-cally slows down the absorption process, which your blood sugar really appreciates. Eating the potato at bedtime has been carefully orchestrated to change your brain chemistry.

Will eating potatoes be bad for my arthritis?

There have been some reports that plants in the nightshade family (which includes potatoes) do make arthritis symptoms flare up. Try a small potato and see if it bothers your arthritis. If it does, use one of the substitutes listed above, but please don't give up on old Mr. Spud without first seeing how it works for you.

If I am going into menopause, should I use sweet potatoes or yams instead?

If you feel this would be valuable for you, you can substitute them for the potato. However, you will lose some of the insulin effect because of the lower glycemic value.

Do I still have to keep eating the potato after I've been on the plan all these months?

Yep. What's more, you don't *have* to keep eating the potato forever and ever, you *get* to. It offers you benefits that you would be foolish to give up. We're not only talking about balancing your brain chemistry, but keeping it balanced. What a concept!!

Your sugar-sensitive biochemistry isn't going to go away. But you can keep it in balance and hold it steady. The spud helps. Don't discard the spud!

Questions on Choosing and Preparing Your Potato

What kind of potato is best to eat?

Any kind of potato is fine, although a mammoth two-pounder may be a little more than you can handle before bed. Choose a spud that suits you. Have fun; explore the wonderful world of potatoes.

Potatoes are classified by shape, skin color, and use. Russets are good for a variety of uses but are best for baking. Rounded or long whites can be used for either boiling or baking, and small red and specialty gourmet potatoes are ideal for boiling. "New" potatoes (small potatoes that are dug early before the skins have set) are best boiled or steamed.

How large or small a potato should I eat?

Experiment until you find what works for you. You could start with a small rose potato, for example. The bottom line is, let your body decide.

There will be many variables that will affect this choice. If you're hungry, eat a big one. If you are a little person, have a small one. Pay attention to the effect and adjust the size to get the results you want. Most of us use a small- to medium-sized red, Yukon Gold, or russet. Be sure to eat the skin, too.

Can I eat the potato with butter, salt, and pepper?

You can have anything that is not protein. Olive oil, salt, pepper, spice, butter, flax oil, salad dressing, mustard, salsa, or curry. Be creative.

Can I use mashed potatoes with butter and milk in them?

Stay away from the milk, because it has protein. You can mash the potato with oat or rice milk, however, and be fine. Make sure your spuds have the skin on them when you mash them.

Can I slice the potato into thick french fries and bake them?

Yes. You can bake them in a toaster oven or regular oven with a little olive oil sprinkled over them. Season with Old Bay seasoning, a blend like Mrs. Dash, or just salt and pepper. They are quite good. One of my favorite ways of frying potatoes is on a non-stick pan with olive oil: Slice them thin and fry them with thin-sliced onions and green peppers. Heavenly!

In fact, there are many, many ways to prepare Mr. Spud. You can make fries like these, you can make a potato casserole or soup and have a little each evening, or you can make potato skins. This does *not* have to be boring. Use your imagination and your cookbook. Ask your friends. Be creative.

Are the eyes of the potato toxic? Should I cut them out?

Eyes are not toxic; however, sprouts are poisonous. Choose potatoes that are well-formed, smooth, and firm, and without discoloration, cracks, bruises, or soft spots. Avoid potatoes with green-tinted skin. Green potatoes have been exposed to light and can have a bitter taste.

Where do you buy purple potatoes?

Many stores that carry organic produce have these now. They are called Peruvian purples. They seem to be more available on the East and West Coasts. But ask your store to get them.

Questions on the Timing of Your Potato

I'm uncertain about when to apply the potato at bedtime since I'm doing the three-meals-a-day plan.

The plan is three meals *and* a baked potato. Eat the potato three hours after dinner and before you go to bed.

Should I wait three hours from the beginning of supper or three hours from the end of supper to eat the potato?

It depends on how long your meal is. The ideal interval for the potato effect is three hours after having protein. Use your own judgment.

I rarely have three hours between dinner and the potato. It's more like one to one and a half hours. Am I wasting my time eating it? (Even at that rate, it still acts like a stimulant and I have trouble falling asleep, and sometimes I feel worse the next day.) If so, should I do the potato/slow carb three hours after lunch instead?

You are either eating really late or going to bed really early. Something is out of sync. Certainly try having the potato after lunch. But the stimulant effect will quiet down in a few weeks and you should be fine.

When I'm at work, I have a tea break at about 5 P.M., but my shift doesn't end until eleven, and then I need to unwind for an hour or so before I sleep. If I eat the potato at about 8 P.M., in the middle of my shift, will I feel mellow and sleepy? Or will I just work away the effects, so it's not as useful? And if I wait until I get home, is it too late to be effective?

I gather you are working the 3 to 11 P.M. shift. Is your tea break for tea or for your evening meal? Eat your meal and have the potato three hours later. You can take Mr. Spud in a plastic bag. The "sleep" effect doesn't seem to kick in until later on when you are in REM dreaming state (about 3 A.M.). You will simply feel more relaxed and focused in dealing with crisis. Spud is not a drug; he's a food! Just relax and make sure you have dinner.

I work/sleep a crazy schedule. Please give me advice/guidance/rules on how to work the potato in.

The practice of figuring out what is right for you is part of your own healing. Sometimes, sugar-sensitive people work and sleep in crazy schedules because they are so out of balance. As they do the food plan, things start to shift. They start actually *planning* on the fact that they need to stop and eat dinner. Or they realize that staying up until 3:00 A.M. to study is crazy. These changes are not psychological but come with the change in brain chemistry.

Work to get three meals with protein at regular intervals. Do the best you can. Come to the Community Forum and ask for help with this. Take a baked spud in a plastic bag with you and eat it even if you are on the run or are eating it at your computer. Things will get better.

What if I can't eat the spud exactly at three hours? Is it okay to eat it one or two hours before or after the three-hour time frame?

The three-hour interval is not absolute, simply ideal. Do the best you can.

Can I eat a raw potato instead of having to cook one?

No, raw potatoes do not give you the effect we are looking for. Raw potatoes are pretty indigestible and have little nutritional value. Cook those spuds!

Is it okay to cook seven potatoes all at once for the whole week?

Many people have found that preparing the potato ahead makes it easier to have one. Others simply pop a spud into the microwave each evening. Find what works for you. But I wouldn't keep leftovers any longer than three days.

Questions on How to Make the Plan Work

Once I eliminate sugar, how long will it take for my mood swings to level off?

The mood swings actually can level off *before* you go off of sugar. Remember, going off sugar is the sixth step of the plan, not the first. Having breakfast with protein, eating the potato at night, and having three meals at regular intervals will all have a positive effect on your mood. Later in the plan, after all those other steps, you do your sugar detox. Once you have completed your sugar detox, you can expect pretty dramatic changes in a week or so.

Is your plan in line with OA (Overeaters Anonymous)?

Absolutely. I attend twelve-step programs and I think they can provide a wonderful support to anyone with a sugar-sensitive body (and therefore an addictive biochemistry). Doing my program and OA together is a pretty unbeatable combination.

I disagree, however, about having to be rigid with rules and about the twelve-step definition of abstinence as *no* slips or you start all over. I prefer a kinder approach that acknowledges the person's commitment to healing.

If I exercise a lot, is it okay to snack?

If you are in training for athletic events or you engage in strenuous physical activity or exercise, it is realistic to add more food into your plan. Try one of the following for between-meal snacks:

- An apple, two cheese sticks, and a handful of almonds
- A baked potato with cottage cheese
- A turkey sandwich on whole grain bread and a pear
- Chinese foods like chicken and broccoli—ask them to hold the MSG and sugar
- Egg salad and a whole grain bagel

Also, you may find that if you have more protein and really complex carbohydrates at your meals, you are less frantic after exercise. If you need a snack during a long run or bike ride, I would try having a George's Shake made with oat milk, which will keep without refrigeration.

What if I can't afford this plan?

People who are homeless and people who are very rich are on this plan. You can definitely design a plan that works for you and your budget.

Fish as a protein does cost more than macaroni and cheese. But don't scare yourself. There are many, many protein foods such as eggs, lentils, kidney beans, chicken thighs, turkey, yogurt, tofu, peanut butter, tuna, and cottage cheese that can work for you if you are on a careful budget.

Also, as you progress with the plan, you won't be buying all sorts of junk food and snack food. Your food budget will stay the same, but what you buy with it will change.

What if I hate to eat alone?

Part of being sugar sensitive is feeling isolated. When we feel isolated and disconnected, doing things alone is harder. Eating alone can be a real drag because you have to buy the food, prepare it, eat by yourself, and then clean up. This is no fun for any of us. Find ways to have meals that are easy to prepare and don't require cleanup. Read a book while eating. Watch TV while eating. I know that all the experts tell you not to do that, but they aren't people who live alone. Create what will work for you, because having three meals a day is really important.

What if I am too busy to cook?

Many of the people I talk to who are succeeding with the program have had to deal with this problem. The most popular solution seems to be to set aside time after grocery shopping to clean and chop vegetables, cook some meats in advance, boil eggs, and so on. That way, when they're caught up in the rush of their day-to-day life, they can open the fridge and grab stuff.

Other folks have done detective work at their local delis and restaurants and come up with lists of things that they can buy there, such as

- Tuna or egg salad sandwiches on whole grain bread
- Caesar salad with grilled chicken
- Fajitas
- Kabobs
- Baked potato with cheese and veggies from the salad bar
- Patty melt on rye
- Chef salad
- Meat- or bean-filled burrito

There's another aspect to this problem that you should consider, however. Being too busy can reflect an unfocused and scattered mind, which is one of the symptoms of low serotonin. You may find that by taking the time to make changes to your food, you end up being able to get everything done—and in significantly less time.

Is taking St. John's wort okay on this plan?

St. John's wort can be a nice addition to the Potatoes Not Prozac Program, but follow directions on dosage and be careful about sun exposure. Also, pay attention to foods that are high in the amino acid tyrosine (such as red wine and aged cheese), because they may cause an adverse reaction. Dr. Michael Murray has great information on the herb in his *Encyclopedia of Natural Medicine.*

People have also asked me about using 5HTP. I am extremely cautious about using supplements for which we have little factual information and whose processing standards are not regulated. By using this supplement, you are cranking up your level of serotonin without letting your body find its own level. As you might guess, my bias is always to use the least harmful method first—that is, eating food rather than taking supplements or medication.

Isn't having a little red wine every day good for the heart?

I have to admit that I have a bias against red wine or any form of alcohol as a way to improve heart health. Red wine acts as a really quick sugar for sugar-sensitive people. The health benefits obtained from red wine can be achieved in other ways. Alcohol is a solvent and achieves its relaxation effects by melting the lipid layer of the brain. For some people a little alcohol is great, but for many of us, it is not so good. I have a great life without alcohol, and I encourage you to do so, too.

Can I drink a George's Shake as a meal twice a day?

Once a day is fine, but please, please don't rely on supplemental foods (even those I recommend) to replace your regular meals. Remember, we are also working toward behavioral changes that include taking care of yourself and fixing yourself real meals. Be cautious with other commercial shake mixes, because they generally have lots of added sugars, often disguised as complex carbohydrates. Read labels. And remember, any shake should contain *both* protein and complex carbohydrate.

What about my comfort foods, like nonfat latte with Sweet'n Low?

Until you have gotten to Step 5, when you switch from browns to whites, you can keep eating your comfort foods, whether they are muffins, chocolate cake, or French bread. In fact, you can continue to eat sugar foods until you have done a sugar detox as part of Step 6. Just eat them with a full meal, *and as you do so,* notice your own emotional attachment to them. See if you can tease out what part of your enjoyment comes from the biochemical response these foods temporarily give you and what part of your enjoyment comes from what you associate with what you are eating. Did your mom bake muffins on Saturday mornings? Did you always have chocolate cake and ice cream for your birthday?

Also, think about what other kinds of foods—nutritious ones—would comfort you. Some folks love hot soup or butternut squash cooked with nutmeg and butter. Also take a look at the recipes at the end of the book. There are several there that might fit the bill, including Cottage Cheese–Cinnamon Pancakes, Pizza with Whole Wheat Crust, Whole Wheat Lasagna, Cornbread, Yam and Cheese Strudel, Pumpkin Cake with Cream Cheese–Peanut Butter Frosting, and Carrot Cake.

As to your vanilla latte with Sweet'n Low, can you substitute an unsweetened decaf latte for it? Or try having a soy latte. I am very leery of the effects of artificial sweeteners.

Finally, consider our trusty friend the potato. When people were asked to rate various comfort foods as to how full and satisfied they felt after eating them (see the box below), the humble potato came out miles ahead!

Food	Rating on the Satiety Index
Potatoes	323
Popcorn	154
Cookies	120
Pasta	119
Jelly beans	118
French fries	116
White bread	100
Ice cream	96
Chips	91
Doughnuts	68
Cake	65
Croissant	47

6

Creating a Routine

Now that you have been working with the program for a while, you need to spend a little time holding steady with your new skills. This may be anywhere from a few weeks to a few months. Steady means firm, unfaltering, unflappable, and unwavering. Steady means driving in cruise control. Steady is what this phase of your program is all about. If you compare this phase of your program to the days before you started, it may seem kind of quiet. The idea of steady may seem boring to you. Let's listen to some friends from the forum.

Here's what Denise writes:

Steady is perseverance with the plan, taking it on faith, and starting to see the light at the end of the tunnel. Steady is believing that this has worked for others and it will work for me because it feels like the right thing to do. Steady is getting back up if I slip because I know this is the direction I want to head in. Steady is not letting myself get sidetracked by frustration and other emotions. Steady is an accumulation of good days!

Phyllis puts it this way:

Steady is how it feels when I'm giving my body the right stuff and staying away from the wrong stuff. It's part of the initial learning stage, where you begin to hear what your body is trying to tell you. You're not off sugar yet, but you are beginning to make the changes that lead to it. As you do so, you begin to feel things differently.

And here is Annette:

Steady is boring—and that's good! I was so accustomed to struggling through my life, I have had to re-evaluate how I look at everyday tasks and events. What happened was that getting stable with my eating and journaling began to open my mind to the possibilities of everyday living. Steady gave me enough clarity to see that I could approach things differently, less emotionally.

Doing Regular Life

Let's review the five things you are working on:

1. Eating three meals with protein at regular intervals
2. Having your potato at night
3. Taking your vitamins
4. Planning your meals and shopping for them
5. Keeping your food journal

At this point in the program, this is *all* you need to do. Five things. One for each finger on your right hand. Nothing more. Do not try to make huge changes to your food right now. Make sure you eat enough. Don't be thinking this is a diet and you need to cut back on your food. You may waver while you are learning new tools. Keep writing in your journal. Keep reading what you have written. Look for patterns, make adjustments, and listen to your body.

Enjoying the Routine

Your whole life you may well have fought against "boring" and yearned for "exciting." I want you to discover a new concept in this phase. If you get your food consistent and stable, your life will start to get more *interesting*. When this happens, the drama that you looked for in making all the changes in what you are eating will come through in your life. You will notice emerging creativity, humor burbling up, positive changes in your job, and changes in your interests—all sorts of things you never thought were connected to what you are eating. It is hard to describe, but it *will* happen.

Tips from the Field: No Fear

My task in life used to be struggling to get past my fears, insecurities, and self-hatred to do what I wanted to do in my life. More often now, my task (my privilege!) is to enjoy observing all the wonders that happen around me, knowing what I want to do, then saying and doing what I feel without fear. I won't kid you and tell you that I feel this every minute of every day, but even when I am feeling cloudy or anxious, I know that it will pass if I continue to "do the food." Miraculous! I love this! This is what it's all about!

—*D.*

Refining the Plan

Getting steady with your plan does not mean making huge changes, it means making small ones. Refinements. For example, maybe you will figure out that dinner works better for you at 6:00 P.M. instead of 7:00 P.M. Or you may find that breakfast at 7:45 A.M. works really well for you. Remember, this is an individualized plan. It's not about getting it right in terms of what I want you to do. It's about getting it right for you, for your rhythm and your body.

Get so steady about doing your meals, food planning, and grocery shopping that you don't have to think about them anymore. They will become automatic. They will become part of the fabric of your life and you won't be thinking about food all the time.

This is the time to just do the program and create the refinements that work for you. But don't mess with the program's basics! Don't ask if you can skip breakfast or have juice instead of a potato. Or have a can of Slim-Fast instead of a George's Shake. Try not to argue about the order of the steps of the program. I have designed them to support your finding your way out of sugar addiction. The steps are the map for your sugar-sensitive body. Eat the potato and keep the journal!

What to Do If You Slip

After you have been steady for a while, you may be distressed to find yourself in a slippery place. You may forget to have breakfast or stop writing in your journal. You may start having a bagel and latte as breakfast or a glass of wine while cooking dinner.

Some people find that while they may slip, they notice it right away and simply get back on track. More often, one slip becomes a little wobble and then the wobble gets bigger and you wake up and realize you aren't feeling so well. The fog has crept back in; you are tired or cranky. Go back to your food journal and take note of what has been going on. You may have thought it was the stress level of your in-laws visiting, but a trip through your journal may tell you that the meal at the restaurant on the evening they arrived started with homemade Italian bread and then went to pasta, wine, and dessert. Maybe what you thought was stress was really all the bread and lack of protein.

The most important thing is kindness and tenderness. All of us, including me, wobble from time to time. It is part of the process. I admit to having a weakness for eggnog lattes. They call me every Christmastime. Part of being steady is being able to notice the wobble and make a correction. If you can go back to your process and your body with humor and tenderness, you may find that the slips give you wonderful information about the most vulnerable places in your program. Use them, learn from them, and build on them.

Check back in your food journal for where you first started to veer off the program. It's likely that smaller slips, like not having enough protein with your breakfast, preceded the big slip that got your attention (say, skipping breakfast for two days and snacking on sugar in mid-afternoon). Or you let more than five or six hours go by between meals. Also, take a look at the feelings you recorded at the time. This program is about listening to your body and learning how what you eat affects both your feelings and your behavior.

Sometimes the start of the slip is not keeping your food journal. As you get steady, you may feel that you "know" what you eat and how you feel. Please, please, please do the journal. It will keep you safe in troubled times and will guide you back when you wander off.

Coming Back After a Full Crash

You may fall off the program big time. Twelve-step people call this relapse. You can call it crashing. You may find that even the idea of giving up sugar and sweet things is propelling you to eat more of them than you used to. This is a natural response to that stress; everybody goes through it. Don't be alarmed. Just keep having three meals a day with protein.

If you do crash, the first thing is, don't beat yourself up.

Learning to stay on the program is part of the healing. No one takes a straight line to the end. The power of your recovery comes with how well you deal with these crashes. Be kind, be gentle, and be firm, too. Take a deep breath and go back to Step 1. Keep it really simple. Just focus on eating breakfast with protein every day. Eat the potato. Journal. Then three meals a day with protein and complex carbs.

The good news is that coming back gets easier each time. You know the drill. If you can keep from criticizing yourself about failure, you will be fine. You have the skills to return to the program and start anew. Use your slips as an opportunity to learn and grow. Over time, you will get steadier and steadier.

Tips from the Field: Compassion in Troubled Times

When my food is off, I am the least clear and compassionate with myself—and this at a time when I need the *most* compassion in order to carry out the detective work and find the source of my crash.

It has been a lesson in letting go of the old self-punishing diet mentality and continuing to grow in compassion. When I slip badly and feel worthless and ashamed, I try to view myself the way a friend would see me—lovingly, forgivingly. Then I go back and highlight parts of my journal and make concrete plans on how to change things.

—A.

Writing in Your Journal Every Day

If you think keeping your journal is boring, it's an important clue. It may mean that you are not using your journal to discover what your body has to say. You may be dutifully logging your food, but not listening to your body.

The value of your journal comes in *using* it. When you really understand that your journal is a way for your body to talk with you, everything will change.

If you see your journal only as a log to record how well (or how poorly) you are doing, it will get old really fast. However, if you work with your journal as a living dialogue with your body, it can be a joy. You will *want* to write in it. You will want to read it and use it to understand what your body needs.

Your body wants to be in relationship with you. It wants to talk with you about how it feels. It wants to teach you what it needs, but it can do so only by giving you its symptoms. Symptoms are the language of your body. If you are feeling better, things are working. If you aren't, you will need to adjust your process and your food. But you can't know the adjustments without your journal.

If you came to my office for a private session, you would bring your journal to research your body's story. These are the questions we would explore together:

- How are you feeling when you wake up? Are you energized? Excited about the day?
- Do you have a hard time waking up? A healthy, rested body wants to get up after sleeping. Even a "night person" will want to get up—albeit more slowly and in increments. When your body is balanced, it is pleased to have another day. If getting up is really hard for you, simply make a note of this. It will change as the food changes.
- When you wake up, do you want to eat breakfast? Are you hungry?
- Are you having breakfast with protein *every* morning? Is this enjoyable?
- Have you developed a breakfast routine that you like? Is it easy and pleasant?

- Has breakfast become automatic and simply a part of your morning without a big hassle?
- Are you having three meals with protein?
- Are you eating enough? Are you eating too much?
- Are you enjoying what you are eating?
- Are you getting the vitamins every day?
- Are you having your evening carbohydrate?

Sometimes people forget the vitamin part. But the vitamins are directly tied in to the processes that convert tryptophan into serotonin. Skip the vitamins and you shortchange your healing. If you will listen, your body will speak to you. Your body has waited through all those years of sugar. It has been forgotten and hidden in shame. Your body wants to talk with you. If you come home to it, your body will respond with a degree of cooperation that will shock you.

Your body loves you. Even if you haven't loved it, it adores you and wants to serve you. It wants to be connected. Spend time; listen to your blessed body. The journal can be your body's voice. Think of that when you read your journal or write in it. Your body has a voice—finally.

Tips from the Field: Learning to Listen

When I first started the program, I did the journal for about a week. Then I forgot about it. But now I am remembering to do it, because *finally* I really want to remember. I really want to hear what is going on in my body and with my food. Before, it was just something I would have to do and which I did not think I needed to do.

—*A.*

No More Fighting—Mastery

This program works really well, but only if you do it. Stop fighting with the program. Worry about the big picture and let go of the tiny little details like how much sugar is in your ketchup. Sugar-sensitive people have a whole lifetime of guilt and shame about their food. More times than they can count, they have tried some new program, resisted it, then given it up—and tried the next new program to come along.

Try to just settle into your routine and master it. It's very simple. Not dramatic. But you do have to do it.

Allowing the Optimism and Feeling Better

Go for gentle optimism as opposed to wild enthusiasm about this program. Wild enthusiasm is what sugar sensitives usually feel when we discover a new program. We think, *Oh my God, I'm gonna do the whole thing. I'm gonna go off sugar, I'm gonna change everything I'm eating, I'm gonna plan my menus, I'm gonna do everything I need to do . . .* Then we end up in the dumps once again—because we can't do it all.

The way to succeed in this program is to just plug away at having three meals a day and eating a potato. Soon you are going to start feeling better and you are going to think, *You know what? Maybe this will work.* Gentle optimism is much more likely to succeed than wild enthusiasm.

Planning Your Food: What's Your Style?

The key to planning your food is to remember that you are not doing *the* Plan, you are doing *your* Plan. And one of the ways you are going to refine the basic plan is to adapt it to your cooking style.

My own style around food is pretty functional these days. I am happy choosing from three or four meal options. It makes my life less complicated. When I was younger I used to cook with energy and enthusiasm. Now, because I have so many other things I want to be doing, I don't really take time to create the kind of fancy meals I once did.

Here are some styles that seem to fit sugar-sensitive people. Take a look and see if one fits you.

The Functional/Factual Type

These people have six choices they use and simply rotate their meals through them. Their foods are simple, relatively un-adorned, and very easy to make. Some functional/factual types have a set for breakfast, a set for lunch, and a set for dinner. They have two eggs, a piece of whole wheat toast, and some juice every morning for breakfast. They eat a tuna sandwich on rye and chips from the lunch truck every day. And for dinner they have the same frozen meal.

The "I Don't Want to Change" Type

These folks eat the same breakfast every day and then vary their other two meals from two or three choices. They like ritual and predictability. They have been eating the same breakfast for ten years. This is a simple approach that works very well with the program.

The One-Pot/One-Meal Type

The one-pot people put everything they are going to have for the day into a stewpot, a casserole dish, or a baking pan. They eat from this pot until it is done, then start again with a new and different concoction. This works fine as long as you don't fish all the protein (chicken, beef, tofu, whatever) out of the pot at your first meal. In fact, you may want to wait to add the protein—say, 4 to 6 ounces of cooked chicken—into each serving you give yourself. That way you know you'll be getting enough.

The Salad Type

The salad folks usually skip breakfast (which we know is not good!), then have all their meals consist of lettuce with different things added to it. These folks can succeed with the program if they don't mind eating salad and protein for breakfast instead of skipping it and if they are willing to accept that lettuce doesn't count as a vegetable (not enough bulk to it). The lettuce can be the backdrop to the real salad of tomatoes, cucumbers, carrots, shredded cabbage, zucchini, red onion, red and green peppers, jicama, celery, cold cooked green beans, broccoli, asparagus, and so on! If you add protein to your salad via hard-boiled eggs, cooked chicken, tuna, anchovies, even cold grilled steak (it's heavenly on a salad!), you'll be fine.

The Eat-on-the-Run Type

These are the people who eat in the car, eat standing up, find something on the fly, and have snacks in the glove compartment. This type can stay on the program if (and only if) they or someone who is taking care of them cooks or buys the food they are going to eat on the run. You cannot successfully eat on the run if you don't pay close attention and *plan* what you are going to eat and when you are going to eat it.

One tip: Pack last night's dinner leftovers in plastic containers and eat them on your way in to work. Or on your way back to your desk after using your lunch hour to work out. Or in the stands at your kid's soccer game. Eating on the run can work if you have access to good food.

The "I Eat If You Fix It" Type

These are the people who eat cereal or cheese and crackers unless someone else makes them a meal. You can only succeed as an "I eat if you fix it" type if you have someone to do the fixing. If you have a good fixer, you will do very well (like Oprah with her personal cook). If you don't, you are in trouble. Eating cereal won't cut it on this plan. You may be able to get by if you have a good deli or supermarket that makes good take-out proteins and things like salads and grilled veggies. But you will have to go get them. And later, when you get further into this program, you will have to be sure there is no sugar in the sauces or salad dressings!

Frankly, if you are this type, I recommend that you choose a new style. Pick the one that is easiest for you and work on it.

The Cooking Type

These are the people who actually use cookbooks and prepare meals. They enjoy it. And the cookers have subtypes ranging from Betty Crocker Miss Homemaker of Tomorrow (that was me in a past life!) to gourmet cooks to just your mother (or your father) in the kitchen. These are the people who read recipes for enjoyment, who like to shop and make meals. If this is your type, you'll sail through this program!

A Little Exercise Always Helps

Everyone tells us we should exercise, right? Right. So there must be a good reason! What they don't always tell you about exercise, though, is that once you get used to it, your body will want to do it. You won't have to use discipline anymore to get yourself walking or bicycling or swimming. Just as you will gradually need less and less self-discipline to eat the right foods for your sugar-sensitive body.

Exercise has an essential role in healing sugar sensitivity. In the first place, it evokes a nice slow rise in your beta-endorphins, those wonderful neurotransmitters that boost your self-esteem and make you feel optimistic, competent, and compassionate—in short, a credit to the human race. What a great feeling! The second key thing that exercise does is make your body more sensitive to insulin. This helps in moving the sugar from your blood into your muscles, where it can be used as fuel. When you are overweight, your body does this less efficiently. Exercise helps to repair this problem.

If you think you can't exercise, see if you can start by committing to exercise *one minute more* a day. If you are doing no exercise now, that means that on your first day you are going to do only one minute. Walk to the end of the driveway and back in one minute. That's it. The next day you are going to add a second minute. Keep going one minute more each day.

If you get up to five minutes, but six minutes seems too long, do five minutes until you feel like you can do six minutes. Do it for three days. Do it for a week if you need to. At some point, you will realize that you *can* do six minutes, and you will. Then keep increasing it one minute at a time. You are aiming for thirty minutes a day. You might need only a month to get there. You might take three months. Slow but steady wins the race. I just started doing this at the gym, and I've gone from five minutes to fifteen minutes in two weeks—with no pain. My body is thrilled.

So the bottom line on exercise is this: It doesn't work if you don't do it. And it works if you do. The key is to start—one minute at a time.

Water, Water All the Time

Drink lots and lots of water. Fill a liter bottle with water and carry it with you. Sip it all day long. Put a slice of lemon in it if you want. Try to have two whole bottles (which equals 64 ounces, or eight glasses of water) each day. If you weigh more than 200 pounds, drink more than that.

I use a rough guideline of drinking half your body weight in ounces of water each day. If you weigh 140, drink 70 ounces of water. If you weigh 240, drink 120 ounces. You may think that if you do this, you will have to pee all day. But a funny thing happens. As your body gets used to more water, your need to pee will be less frantic. If you're over fifty and having problems with urinary incontinence, it actually will get *better* over time as you increase your daily water intake. If you are exercising, it will get better even more quickly.

Our bodies love having plenty of water. Water carries nutrients to our cells, carries toxins back out of them, and keeps our skin moist. In addition, it aids in the working of neurotransmitters like serotonin and beta-endorphin. Our brain functions with electricity. Water conducts electrical signals. If our brain is dehydrated, the electrical signals won't get transmitted properly. Drink water.

Remember, increase your water intake, not just your fluid intake. Juices, coffee, milk, tea, and soda *do not count* as water. In fact, coffee, tea, and cola are diuretics and make your body *lose* water. If you do drink them, in addition to your 8 to 10 glasses of water a day, drink an additional 12 ounces, for example, for each 12-ounce can of soda.

Many sugar-sensitive people have a hard time remembering to drink more water. "I just am not thirsty," they say. It seems that for many people, the thirst signal, like the hunger signal, doesn't work the way it should. You don't notice thirst until you are in big trouble. Drink water by the clock rather than by your thirst. And note in your food journal how much water you have had for the day.

Tips from the Field: Water, Everywhere

I treated our family to an in-home water cooler so we have cold water on hand all the time. They drink more, I drink more. I also keep a couple half bottles of water in the freezer, so when I need to go out for the day, I fill the bottle of ice to the top with water and it stays cold for the rest of the day.

—*M.*

Why Some Stuff Will Help

My readers have suggested a number of kitchen appliances that can help you find the road to steady. People started to spontaneously vote for their favorites. Here are the appliances that were voted tops by our community.

Indoor Grills

These are little grills that open up and allow you to place your food between the grill plates. They were originally designed as "lean meat" machines because they are shaped to let the fat drain off. But they are easy to use and clean and make the food taste great. They got the majority vote.

Toaster Oven

Toaster ovens can handle many, many tasks, ranging from cooking the spud to reheating yesterday's leftovers or cooking a frozen dinner. They are easy to use and a great resource for turning a cold meal into a hot dinner.

Crock-Pot

The one-pot people all know the miracle of the Crock-Pot. The rest of you will be delighted to discover that hot chili can be waiting to eat right when you get home from work. No waiting, no cooking, just sit down and eat. Chili, soup, stew, beans, roasts—you name it; the one-potters make it.

Rice Cooker

Sometimes you shy away from making real rice—long-grain brown rice—because you feel it takes too long. You really have to keep an eye on it so the pot doesn't boil over and slop that wet rice stuff down into the burner pan. A rice cooker lets you set it up, then go take care of the rest of your life while you are waiting for dinner. And the rice comes out perfect every time.

Blender

Ah, the joys of the blender. Use the blender to mix your George's Shake for breakfast. Use the blender to make something quickly if you are over the cliff. Every sugar-sensitive kitchen needs a blender.

Your Oven

A shocking thought—cook food in the oven! Make a roasted chicken, putting two potatoes in the pan along with a pound of cut up carrots, and voilà! Dinner in an hour—no hassle. And those potatoes baked in the oven taste mighty fine.

Use Your Freezer

If you make good use of your freezer, you can cook once a week and have things to eat all week long. Store individual portions in plastic bags. No preparation needed, just heat it up and eat. Make your own TV dinners.

Trying New Foods—Starting to Explore

Many sugar sensitives know how to make only bread, muffins, cookies, brownies, and good things like that—you tend to be masters at making "white things." It's time to learn to grill a steak, roast a chicken, make fabulous salad dressing, stir-fry veggies, and sauté cabbage (then bake it in sour cream). Be outrageous. Go to the grocery store and try something new every week. Ask your friends who cook (you might have one or two who do) to teach you about new foods. Take a cooking class.

Veggies Are for Real

When you think of vegetables, do you groan and make a face? Does the thought of broccoli make you ill? Many sugar-sensitive people feel (or used to feel) that way. You remember being told that you couldn't leave the dinner table until you ate the lima beans. Couldn't have dessert until you'd at least *tried* the cauliflower au gratin. And now that you are adults and can control (or think you can) what you put in your mouths, the only vegetables you eat are french fries, iceberg lettuce, and sometimes corn.

Tips from the Field: Veggie Detente

You can change your relationship to vegetables! I grew up eating no veggies. There was always semi-moldy iceberg lettuce in the refrigerator. I, like President Reagan, counted ketchup as a vegetable. I guess I have a "kid's appetite" in not liking vegetables. But I have friends (many) who LOVE veggies.

Since being on the program, I have tried to add more veggies to my food plan. I started off for a few months having 3 to 5 veggies PER MONTH (no kidding!) I actually got up to one veggie per day, which is great for me. I can't say I got to the point where I love them, but I definitely improved.

—*L.*

The best suggestion for people who dislike veggies is to cook once (or twice) for the week. One week, for example, you could buy a prime rib roast marinated in garlic that might give you five or six meals. Cook lots of vegetables (carrots, onions, and potatoes with skins) with the roast. You'll find yourself *loving* those vegetables! The garlic helps.

Use the leftovers to design different "quick" meals. Mix some of the meat with brown rice and veggies in a stir-fry; or top a whole wheat pizza with some of the meat shredded on top of the cheese.

You can also cook a meatloaf and eat it for the week. You sneak veggies into your meatloaf. Grated carrots, green and red peppers, peas, anything you can find. One of my clients had a "meatloaf marathon," and made three different kinds of meatloaf. (See Chapter 11 for numerous recipes.) She froze two of the kinds of meatloaf and ate the third until it was almost gone. Then she defrosted the second and ate it. She said it was fun, and because of the different recipes, she never got bored.

Great Vegetables to Get Started With	
Cooked	*Raw*
Carrots	Carrots
Peas	Red peppers
Butternut squash	Yellow peppers
Corn	Jicama
Yams	Mushrooms

Here's another idea for getting started with vegetables. Begin with the sweeter varieties. Your sugar-sensitive tongue will like them better. Take a look at the vegetables in the box above. Don't even think of starting with lima beans or brussels sprouts. They will scare you. Start with the vegetables that seem friendly to you.

Another way to make vegetables tastier is to melt cheese (cheddar, Jack, even Gouda) on top of them or use a sauce. One of my broccoli-loathing friends actually ate a dish of lightly cooked broccoli and cauliflower covered with a peanut-soy sauce that he found in a Japanese cookbook. The flavor of the sauce was strong enough to tone down the flavor of the veggies.

Another really helpful thing to try is to go to the farmer's market and get fresh vegetables. You will not believe the difference in taste between a brussels sprout from the stalk in late November and those nasty ones that come frozen in boxes.

Tips from the Field: Making Friends with Veggies

I try to cut up fresh veggies and leave them in the fridge to grab. I eat them more often if they don't have to be cut and cleaned each time. I also hard-boil a few eggs to leave in the fridge to eat when I need that quick protein boost.

—*T.*

I blanch my veggies by submerging them in boiling water for a minute or two, and then I make them into salads with dressings. I use broccoli, zucchini, green beans, red and green peppers, and spuds. My favorite dressing is mustard mixed with mayonnaise. I also toss blanched or raw veggies into quiche, egg salad, or baked potatoes. I nearly always have coleslaw with mayonnaise in the fridge. Sometimes I just add the raw veggies to that. I love my veggies now, but I used to struggle with them big-time.

—*S.*

Trying New Recipes

The next time you are in a bookstore or library, browse through the cookbooks. See if you can find one that appeals to you. If you are fairly new to cooking, keep it simple! Don't try gourmet cookbooks or elaborate recipes for foreign foods. Stick to the cookbooks for quick or easy-to-make meals. There's even a cookbook out there that is devoted entirely to recipes that require only three ingredients. Take a look at kids' cookbooks, too. The directions are simple, and the recipes are usually pretty yummy.

Ask Your Friends for Best Recipes

Don't do this recipe stuff alone! Your friends may have favorite simple recipes that they love. Ask them! Stress that you are not looking for recipes fit for the queen of England, but for someone (you) who wants a few new, easy ideas for putting meals on the table. Remember that people who love to cook also love to share what they do.

Planning for Downtimes

It's inevitable. There will be times when you are on the run and can hardly remember your name, let alone your food plan for the day. Ironically enough, the key to handling these danger times is to plan for them. If you know you will have a meeting through lunch, bring something with you to have before the meeting. Know the meal choices in your local convenience store so that the raisins or candy bars don't hop into your mouth while your blood sugar has crashed and you are falling off the cliff.

Stocking Your Cupboards

Remember this idea from Chapter 3? It is *important.* It works. If you haven't done it yet, go back to page 59 and read this section again. Get your basics in place. Don't be skipping the early stuff because you think it doesn't apply to you.

I make sure I have some core foods on hand. My list includes ground meat, chicken breasts, canned tuna, frozen salmon, eggs, cheese, cottage cheese, natural peanut butter, almonds, potatoes, oatmeal, rye crackers, frozen veggies, and bananas. This means that when I forget the time and haven't planned, I always have something on hand to use for dinner.

Tips from the Field: What Not to Run Out Of

I quite often cook the meats ahead and microwave the rest. I use one of those plastic divided plates. I fill up the plate from my bags of frozen veggies, precooked meats, leftover skin-on mashed potatoes, and so on.

Even if I don't have any precooked meat or leftover potatoes, at least I can fill my plastic plate with frozen veggies straight from the bag, add a dash of olive oil, salt and pepper, and grab a can of tuna.

—D.

When You Crash and Don't Know What to Do

If you skipped lunch and it's 4:00 P.M., you may figure out that you are in trouble. But sometimes sugar-sensitive people actually need to eat more than they let themselves when they are in diet mode. They may think they are doing everything right, but they often don't eat enough lunch and by mid-afternoon are really foggy or cranky—way beyond being hungry. I call this falling off the cliff. It is a sign of a serious drop in blood sugar. It has a desperate quality to it: You have to eat something right now!

These are the times you reach for sugar. These are the times an alcoholic in early recovery will grab something to drink. You have to have a plan in place before you get to this point. This is sort of like having a fire drill with your kids. You teach them how to get from the bed to the window. You have them practice going down the fire ladder. You don't wait until there is a fire to do the drill.

So in preparation for an over-the-cliff emergency, keep a high protein/low sugar bar in your dashboard. Keep a box of Triscuits under the car seat. You can always scout up some cheese sticks and have a good snack on hand. Know where the fast food places are. Know the choices so you don't have to think. It's a good idea to keep a list handy (maybe in your car) of foods that you can find in your local convenience store when you can't stop for a meal and are desperate for something to eat. The key is that your food needs to include protein. Don't reach for Fritos and a Coke. Here are some suggestions of what you might choose from the convenience store:

- Mozzarella cheese sticks, Triscuits, and milk or V8 juice
- Slices of lunch meat (ham, turkey, bologna, etc.) wrapped around sticks of mozzarella or string cheese and milk or V8 juice
- Hot dogs and V8
- Burrito heated in the store's microwave and milk
- Peanuts, cashews, or sunflower seeds, an apple or orange (if they stock any fresh fruit), and milk or V8
- Triscuits and bean dip with milk or V8
- Mozzarella sticks, corn chips, and salsa
- Triscuits spread with peanut butter and milk

When You Get Hit with the 9:00 P.M. Munchies

Ah, the munchies. This is the time to stop and listen to your body. What are you actually feeling? Are you truly hungry, or are you feeling tired or having withdrawal from the sweet things you had at lunchtime? Are you bored and on the prowl? Write whatever you notice in your journal and see if you can sort it out.

Then go eat your nightly potato. If you're bored, put salsa on it. Or make a hot potato salad by steaming, then slicing your potato and tossing it with your favorite salad dressing.

Foods to Carry With You

It helps a lot if you keep some food with you, either at work or in your car in case of emergency hunger. Here are some of the things folks on the plan have kept handy:

- A box of Triscuits or other whole grain crackers. (These will fill you up and feel more satisfying than crackers made with white flour.) Don't forget to add some protein to your crackers.
- Nuts such as raw or roasted peanuts, almonds, and pecans. Pick a kind you *really* like so you'll feel emotionally satisfied when you need to grab a handful.
- Sandwich spreads that don't need to be refrigerated, such as peanut butter or those funny little cans of deviled ham you may remember from your childhood.
- Salad dressings that don't need to be refrigerated. My favorite is vinaigrette made with sherry vinegar. When I grab a chef salad at a fast food place and pour my special dressing on top, it turns into a yummy lunch.
- Some George's Shake mix packed into a big plastic glass with a lid so you can add juice or milk, shake, and drink!

Tips from the Field:
Protein to Ward Off Hunger Pangs

I used to have a problem with getting hungry at 11:00 A.M. and 3:30 P.M. Then I discovered that if I used *two* scoops of protein powder in milk instead of one after I eat my morning oatmeal, the problem is solved. The hunger doesn't come until lunchtime. The less milk I use, the better this works.

—B.

What to Do If You Miss Lunch Away from Home

This is not the time to beat yourself up or grab a candy bar; this is the time to get thee to a fast food place or a restaurant. At McDonald's you can always get eggs with bacon and potatoes or a grilled chicken salad or chef salad. Other fast food places offer baked potatoes, such as Wendy's spud topped with cheese and broccoli. You could also get Wendy's taco salad and put the chili on the potato. Make your own mental list of the places in your neighborhood that will support you in a crunch. I go to the local New Mexican restaurant and order huevos rancheros—eggs and beans and chili. Does it every time.

7

Halfway There: Step 5

You have been working on the foundation of the Sugar Addict's Total Recovery Program: eating three meals a day with protein, eating them at regular intervals, taking the vitamins, drinking lots of water, and exercising daily. By now, you are probably pretty steady on doing those things as well as keeping your food journal, regularly planning your meals, and going grocery shopping with a list. You have mastered important parts of the program and are ready for taking things out.

This next step will firm up this foundation and get you all set for starting to cut down on sugars. It is about substituting whole grains for the white-flour products you now eat. As you'll see, there is a huge (and delicious) variety of whole grain breads, muffins, cereals, pastas, waffles, and even tortillas on the market today.

Step 5. Shift from White Foods to Brown Foods

One of the simplest ways to grasp this step is to see yourself shifting from eating white things to brown things. It is easy to remember these simple images as you make your food choices. White things are white because the grain or rice they are made from has been refined to remove its brown part, which—ironically—is also the nutrition-packed and fiber-rich part. Food processors do this because they think white things are more visually attractive. They are also sweeter, without fiber to slow down their absorption, so white things are absorbed into your bloodstream much faster than brown things—almost as fast as straight sugar. They cause your blood sugar to spike and set you up for a big fall, both biochemically and emotionally. (A potato eaten with its skin is a brown thing. Eaten without its skin—as most french fries are prepared—it's a white thing.)

Here are some examples of white things. Check off the ones that you regularly eat:

_____ Bagels	_____ Macaroni
_____ White bread	_____ Noodles
_____ Cake	_____ Pancakes made with white flour
_____ Cereal	_____ Pasta
_____ Cookies	_____ Pastry
_____ Crackers	_____ Pie
_____ Croissants	_____ Waffles
_____ Flour tortillas	_____ White rice

How many did you check? I would have checked all of them before I changed my own eating patterns. Sugar-sensitive people _love_ white things—sometimes even more than ice cream or other sweet treats. When you eat them, you want more. For some folks, these addictive foods are the obvious ones, like chocolate, ice cream, cookies, French bread. For others, the foods that call to them are pasta, milk, popcorn, cheese, chips, even Diet Coke.

As diverse as these foods are, they all have a soothing emotional effect. They make you feel safe, comfortable, and loved through their taste or feel or the emotional cues attached to them. Eating them provides you with a safe haven that draws you to them again and again. But they also create havoc in your body and your brain.

You may get spooked by the thought of not eating white things anymore. White things are the foods that most often represent love and comfort. You cannot imagine life without macaroni or white bread. Be gentle with yourself. Take a deep breath. No one is going to take away your favorite foods. The idea is for you to *move toward* using more brown things, to shift toward using them more often, but the shift happens as gradually as you feel comfortable having it happen.

The World of Whole Grains

Nowadays, food manufacturers are heeding the words of nutrition advocates and are starting to offer brown breads, bagels, waffles, crackers, pita bread, and more. Whole grains not only help keep your blood sugar level stable; they also give your body a solid, consistent fuel to draw from.

You will need to do some work to learn which foods are indeed whole grain. Sometimes breads that appear to be brown are actually refined white flour with brown color added. The clue is the weight of the bread or grain. Fiber is heavy. So if you pick up a loaf of bread that looks brown but is as light as Wonder Bread, make another choice. And always read the labels.

Brown Things

Brown things include foods higher in fiber, such as whole grains, seeds, and beans. Here are some examples of what I call brown things.

Whole grain bread

Whole grain cereal

Whole grain pasta

Whole grain pancakes

Whole grain tortillas (corn
   or whole wheat)

Granola, no sugar added

Brown rice

Oatmeal

Sunflower seeds

Potatoes with skin

Sweet potatoes

Refried beans

Kidney beans (used in chili)

Black beans

Garbanzo beans (chickpeas)

Hummus

Lentils

Millet

Pumpkin seeds

Quinoa

Soybeans

Polenta

Yams

I have included some choices that also have protein in them (such as beans and lentils). If you are a vegetarian, you will be counting these as part of your protein. But if you are looking for slow carbohydrates, the bean things will work well. They are hearty, nutritious, and comforting.

Many of these foods you can find in your supermarket. Others you may have to buy at a health food store. As you shift from eating white things to brown things, you'll start noticing big changes in your sense of well-being and your energy level. When you look at your food journal, you will see the connection between your new way of eating and your feelings. You may remember the difference between having optimal or low blood sugar. Brown things support optimal blood sugar levels.

If it is hard to make the shift from white to brown, start by having your white things only with a meal. Try giving up your snack of cinnamon-sugar toast mid-afternoon and have it for lunch. *Make change at the pace that works for you.* Go slowly enough that you don't get spooked, but make change. Work toward solid long-term success, not dramatic short-term results.

Balanced Blood Sugar	Low Blood Sugar
Energetic	Tired all the time
Tired when appropriate	Tired for no reason
Focused and relaxed	Restless, can't keep still
Clear	Confused
Good memory	Trouble remembering things
Able to concentrate	Trouble concentrating
Able to problem-solve effectively	Easily frustrated
Easygoing	More irritable than usual
Even-tempered	Gets angry unexpectedly

This step may be hard. You love white things because they represent comfort and love. Pie at Thanksgiving is the center of the celebration. But as you do your homework and progress through this recovery program, you are going to find ways to keep the positive emotional attachment to the foods that are good for you and let go of the problem foods. It may seem like an impossible dream now, but it will happen! You can have whole wheat or brown rice pasta and be fine. You can have a whole grain bagel instead of a croissant and have all the emotional enjoyment of the ritual. You can make a birthday cake with whole wheat flour that may actually even taste better than the traditional yellow/white cake you usually make. (You might want to bake any recipe made with substitutes before the big day to make sure you don't end up with a disaster that tastes like cardboard.) This shift from white to brown does not have to create panic. It just takes practice.

A Thousand Types of Bread

As I mentioned earlier, most store-bought bread contains refined white flour even though the bread is labeled "brown" or "whole grain." As you read the food label, look for the amount of fiber. Look for 2 or more grams of fiber in each serving. More fiber means more brown.

Also read the label to see if there is sugar added to the bread. It is a common misperception that yeast needs added sugar in order to make dough rise, but yeast can use the sugars already in the flour just fine. Keep looking until you find a bread that is made without sugar. Many of my readers have discovered the joy of making their own bread. Check out some of the recipes in Chapter 11. Try them and discover that brown can be a mighty fine alternative to white.

Tips from the Field: An Alternative to Wheat

I have been using spelt flour and spelt products in place of white flour. I add the flour to whole grain pancake mix for pancakes or waffles, and use it in cornbread batter. My local health food market also carries spelt tortillas and various spelt breads.

—J.

Cereal Options

When you are slowly shifting your food from white things to brown things, don't forget that this shift applies to your morning cereal as well! White cereals include Rice Krispies, Cocoa Puffs, Count Chocula, Frosted Flakes—all the things your children want and you eat at night in front of the TV.

Brown cereals are the boring ones. Here are some examples:

Oatmeal (unsweetened)
Other hot cereals like millet and oat bran and buckwheat
All-Bran (Kellogg's)
Shredded Wheat

If you aren't ready for "full" brown, start by shifting to the cereals that are lower in sugars, like Grape-Nuts and Cheerios (not Honey Nut Cheerios). Look for cereals that have less than 10 grams of sugar per serving.

Have your children help you on this treasure hunt. When you decide to switch cereals, be careful to read the nutrition labels. Many cereals, like breads, are labeled "all natural" and look brown, but they are filled with sugars. Even though we are not focusing on cutting back on sugars in this step, why *add* something sweet to your diet that you'll need to take away later? Commercially made granola is often like this. It sure looks good for you, but it has grams and grams of sugar. Or it has huge amounts of dried fruit added, which is concentrated sugar. Do not use dried fruit, but you can use some fresh or frozen fruits in moderation. Do not use sweetened frozen fruit.

Some natural foods stores now carry unsweetened granola. Granola is a wonderful cereal option to learn to make. You can make it without sugar (or honey) and have a delicious, chewy option for breakfast. I often take a whole grain granola and cook it to make a hearty serving for breakfast. It has a wonderful nutty flavor and is very comforting. You can adapt almost any granola recipe by simply taking out the sugars—things such as honey, brown rice syrup, raisins, and other dried fruits.

Oatmeal: The Wonder Food

Oatmeal is a wonder food because oatmeal has it all: it's inexpensive and easy to cook; it has protein, soluble fiber, no cholesterol, and no sugar; and it is low in sodium. Oatmeal will not only help to maintain your optimal blood sugar level, it will minimize your cravings. You can add protein powder to it or eat it with eggs for a solid breakfast. You can put cinnamon, nutmeg, fruit, and/or milk on it. The Scots add milk and butter, which tastes yummy. You can cook it in milk, soy milk, or apple juice instead of water.

When you buy oatmeal, look for whole grain oats. These are also known as steel-cut oats or Irish oatmeal, and they are the best kind for you. You can toast them lightly in the oven or in a frying pan on the top of the stove before cooking; this changes the flavor to an interesting nutty taste. Whole oats take much longer to cook. They are the top of the "slow" list. If you don't have that much time, use regular rolled oats. Even instant oatmeal will do in a pinch, but stay away from the flavored ones that are chock full of sugars. Try putting butter, salt, and milk on your oatmeal rather than brown sugar. You may really like the Scottish way.

Tips from the Field: Getting Creative with Oatmeal

I fix my oatmeal ahead of time and put each portion in a separate microwavable container. Then, in the morning, I just pop the container in the microwave and it's ready in 3 minutes. I stir in some milk, peanut butter, almonds, and protein powder. Read the directions on the box for the best cooking time.

—M.

I use McCann's Irish oatmeal and dress it up with butter, cinnamon, nutmeg, a splash of vanilla, 1 tablespoon ground flaxseed, a heaping tablespoon of sunflower seed for flavor, crunch, and added protein, and a little bit of either blueberries or strawberries. I can cook the oats while I'm in the shower, and by the time I am finished, they are ready to be doctored up. I love the texture and the flavor, and they hold me over to lunch better than the quick oats.

—C.

I like my (precooked) oatmeal heated in the skillet with the egg mixed in, and a little spray margarine and salt and pepper, sort of like a Scottish matzo brie. On Sundays I cook up two batches of McCann's slow-cooking oatmeal. Then each morning I either nuke and season a serving of it or fry it in a little margarine/butter. Then I scramble an egg, pour it over the oatmeal, and mix the whole thing up.

—J.

Try oatmeal with cottage cheese mixed in. First make the oatmeal, then add the cottage cheese. You may have to heat it some more if you want the cheese to melt. Add some cinnamon and nutmeg, too!

—B.

I make plain instant oatmeal every morning (no sugar). Right when I add the boiling water I mix in a tablespoon of cashew butter (or sugar-free peanut butter). Then I add a chopped apple and a sprinkle of cinnamon. I get my protein, fruit, and complex carbohydrate all in one satisfying tasty bowl.

—A.

For a filling breakfast, I put 4 egg whites in a bowl and microwave them for one minute. Then I stir the egg whites, add ½ cup uncooked oatmeal, stir again, and microwave another minute or until cooked. I also sprinkle some raw nuts such as walnuts or cashews on top and a little nutmeg.

—S.

Pasta Alternatives

Many people have found solace in using whole wheat or brown rice pasta. Don't use the green pastas, because they are simply regular white pasta with spinach added. If you do use the brown pastas and find yourself craving more and more, you need to stop using them. When I eat whole wheat pasta, I start dreaming about a thousand different ways to have it. If I use brown rice pasta, however, it is a nice, comforting, satisfying meal and I have no craving for more. Listen to your own body to know what is right for you.

Don't Forget the Potato!

Don't let the extra effort it takes to shift away from eating white things distract you from the importance of your nightly potato. That humble potato is helping your brain manufacture more serotonin, which will set the stage for the important change to come: cutting down on sugars. With plenty of serotonin, you will approach this otherwise scary step confidently and creatively. An optimal level of serotonin will also lower your cravings for sugar and will actually *increase* your appetite for healthy foods.

You can vary the type of potato you use; you can eat less than a whole one or choose a little one. If you find yourself having wild dreams or insomnia after trying out the potato, have a smaller one. The wild dreams are a sign of the activation of your serotonin system; they mean the potato is working. You need it, but you may need less than what you have been eating. If you are very low in serotonin, you will get a bigger effect from the potato.

Some people just don't like the idea of the potato and will never eat one. Others are allergic to potatoes or potatoes aggravate their arthritis. I try to be realistic. While the potato is best, if you just can't or won't do it, I am willing to negotiate an alternative.

Choose a different slow carb. Try Triscuits or a sweet potato or oatmeal or whole wheat toast or an apple. Just remember not to add anything with protein in it or you will defeat the biochemical purpose of your bedtime carb.

Sometimes people get scared about calories and they skip the evening potato. Think of the evening potato as medicine. Food as pharmacology. The potato (three hours after dinner) is the very thing that is going to help you be able to say no to the things you don't want to eat anymore. It will reinforce your sense of being steady or having discipline.

Have It Your Way, But Have It

The wonderful people on our online Community Forum have come up with lots of creative ways to cook their bedtime potato. Here are some of their simpler suggestions:

- Slice and bake on an oiled cookie sheet to make oven fries (it's a lot faster if you have already cooked the potato).
- Grate it with some onion and fry it up, like hash browns.
- Use leftover mashed potatoes (with skins) to make potato pancakes.
- Cube your potato and microwave it.
- Try any of the above with red potatoes, white potatoes, Yukon Gold potatoes, or Peruvian (purple) potatoes. Also, some folks swear that organic baking potatoes taste much better than the regular russets. (They're also smaller.)
- Rub butter or margarine on the outside of your baking potato to get a wonderfully crispy skin.

How to Have Fun When You Get Bored with Mr. Spud

This is the time to dig out your cookbooks, ask your friends for ideas, and poke around in the library or on the Web for new and unusual recipes. I have found several potato cookbooks. The only restriction on fixing the bedtime potato is that the recipes must not include protein. Even if your new recipe calls for peeling the potatoes, don't do it! You need that brown skin to make your nighttime snack a brown thing!

Oven-Fried Sweet Potatoes

This is a recipe for one person, suggested by Cheryl, a reader. Try this as your before-bed potato. If you want to make these as part of a meal, figure one potato per person.

   1 sweet potato
      Vegetable oil
      Salt and pepper to taste
      Onion powder to taste
      Garlic powder to taste

Wash and peel the potato, then cut it into french-fry-size pieces.
Put a little oil on a cookie sheet or in the tray of your toaster oven,
and dump the fries on it. Turn them to coat all sides with
oil. Then sprinkle with salt, pepper, onion powder, and a little
garlic powder. (Or substitute nutmeg for onion and garlic
powders.)

- If you are using a conventional oven, bake at 450° F. for 15
  minutes, turning once so the bottoms don't burn.
- If you are using a toaster oven, bake at 425° F. for 20 minutes,
  turn them (the bottoms get nicely brown), then turn off
  the oven and let them sit for another 10 minutes.

Ten Toppings for Your Baked Potato
   1. Olive oil
   2. Salsa (try several varieties)
   3. Salad dressing (not blue cheese)
   4. Chives
   5. Mustard
   6. Toasted onion
   7. Pesto
   8. Butter
   9. Pepper
   10. Curry

What to Eat in This Phase

Now that you have mastered Mr. Spud, let's go back to the bigger picture. The white-to-brown shift is not all that hard to do

logistically. It's a good time to try experimenting a little with what you are having. Take another look at your breakfast and lunch menus. These may have included some white or sweet foods as you were learning the routine of breakfast every day. By now they should be including brown things as the carbohydrate part. Let's look at some good ideas that have come from *Potatoes Not Prozac* readers. These are folks just like you who are trying new foods and sharing their new adaptations. Let's see our revised breakfasts first.

Ten Breakfast Ideas from the Field

Earlier in this chapter we talked about brown cereals you could have for breakfast, including several delightful things you could do with oatmeal. Here are some other ideas from folks in our Community Forum. (An asterisk indicates that the recipe is in Chapter 11.)

1. Crustless Quiche* with whole grain toast
2. Yogurt Ricotta Delight
3. Brown rice (leftover rice works fine) fried with two eggs
4. Oatmeal with Grape-Nuts, raisins, and peanuts (optional: add protein powder and cinnamon)
5. Miso soup with tofu, seaweed, green onions, and bean sprouts
6. An egg-and-cheese burrito in a whole wheat tortilla
7. A whole grain waffle with protein powder in the batter, applesauce and plain yogurt on the top
8. Cottage Cheese–Cinnamon Pancakes*
9. Split pea soup and whole grain toast
10. One cup chili served over brown rice

Five Fast Dinners for the Ridiculously Busy

1. Barbecued or roast chicken (bought from the deli), frozen green beans with almonds (5 minutes in microwave), brown basamati rice (reheated from the big batch you cooked on the weekend)

2. A whole wheat tortilla with refried beans and cheese (and leftover chicken or beef if you have it around), nuked for about 45 seconds, and served with sour cream and salsa
3. Scrambled eggs with sliced tomatoes and whole grain toast
4. Brown rice spaghetti, crumbled hamburger in tomato sauce, and frozen corn
5. Sautéed tofu and garlic, steamed broccoli, and a potato baked in the microwave

Five Elegant Dinners

Cooking lavish dinners for company (or for yourself!) is no problem on the food plan. Try these menus—complete with appetizers or soup, main course and desserts—or invent your own, substituting brown things for white things wherever possible.

This is a great menu for a festive winter dinner:

- Roast Sticky Chicken*
- Larry's Famous Green Beans*
- Sweet Potato Puff*
- Whole grain biscuits

Here's a dinner with an oriental flavor:

- Asian Salad*
- Grilled salmon steaks served with lemon wedges
- Stir-Fried Lemon Asparagus*
- Fried Brown Rice with Onions, Almonds, and Cumin*
- Pumpkin Tofu Cheesecake*

Try this summer dinner when artichokes are in season:

- Feta Frittata*
- Jumbo shrimp sautéed in garlic and olive oil, served on a bed of brown basamati rice

- Steamed artichoke with mayonnaise seasoned to taste with curry powder
- Salad of baby organic mixed greens served with vinaigrette made with balsamic vinegar
- Carrot Cake*

This could be a Thanksgiving feast!

- Roast Chicken with Garlic*
- Oven-Fried Sweet Potatoes*
- Peas with mint
- Brown rice and wild rice cooked (separately) in chicken broth and/or beef broth and mixed before serving
- Squash Pie with Peanut Butter Glaze*

Here's a good one for folks who like their food plain and simple:

- Chicken Roasted with Garlic*
- Roasted Potatoes*
- Apple Carrots*
- Fresh-baked whole wheat bread
- Fruit salad with a dollop of plain yogurt, topped with roasted almonds, whole or sliced

One-Pot Meals

- Ratatouille cooked with slices of turkey sausage, ground beef, or chicken. Serve over brown rice, if desired.
- Beef Stew*
- Feta Frittata*
- Chili Layered Casserole*
- Asian Salad*

Your Friends the Vegetables

Many sugar-sensitive people are not all that fond of vegetables and drift to the white side of the grocery store rather than the vegetable side. But you need to get to know the vegetable options. Start with the ones that seem most familiar or with a vegetable you love. Try having it fresh and see the difference. You could even do something really outrageous and get some peas to shell. Put the fresh peas in your salad.

Corn on the cob is an easy vegetable to love. Try it combined with chopped sweet red peppers and steamed young green beans. Or get peeled, cubed fresh squash at the grocery store. Steam it and serve sprinkled with grated cheese and nutmeg—you will be stunned at how good it is. Try grilling veggies that you have brushed with olive oil on the barbecue grill—on skewers or not or on your lean, mean grilling machine. Peppers, onions, carrots, mushrooms, and zucchini slices taste entirely different when grilled.

Stir-fry your veggies in olive oil. Get a package of ready-to-stir-fry fresh vegetables at the grocery story. Cook them so that you can stick a fork in them, but don't let them get mushy. Sprinkle them with onion salt or roasted garlic.

Try eating your vegetables raw; put them in your salad. Arrange them on your plate. Play with your food. Be bold!

Finding New Comfort Foods

Now that you're shifting away from foods made with white flour, you may need to pick some other foods to substitute for comfort foods like pasta, bagels, French bread, and doughnuts. There are two ways to go with this. Sometimes it is easy enough to substitute the whole grain version of the food for the white version, such as substituting whole grain bagels or waffles or pizza dough for the kind made with white flour, or swapping Triscuits for Ritz crackers, which are made of whole wheat. Take care that you don't develop cravings for the whole grain foods. Another option is to see if entirely different foods can provide comfort when you need it. Some of these foods might be soups like cream of chicken or split pea, dishes like chili, quiche, frittata, burritos (on whole wheat tortillas), Yam and Cheese Strudel, or Sweet Potato Pie (recipes for these two are in Chapter 11).

Sometimes the comfort comes from the ritual surrounding having the food. I used to *love* pizza—not so much for the pizza as for the treat. Pizza meant not having to cook. Pizza meant sharing with friends, being goofy, the smell of the pizza place, and of course the cold beer with it. I don't go into pizza places even now because all the sounds and smells trigger a desire for pizza. But I do make an adapted pizza to eat at home, and that works just fine. The recipe is in Chapter 11.

Let's take a look at how you feel about your own comfort foods. In the space below, write down your current comfort foods. Then write down what you might have instead—for example, bran muffins or Oatmeal Muffins (recipe in Chapter 11) instead of blueberry muffins. You may need to make a trip to your grocery or natural foods store to see what your whole grain options are. There are more than you think!

Old Comfort Foods	*New Comfort Foods*
_____	_____
_____	_____
_____	_____
_____	_____
_____	_____
_____	_____

Unfortunately, there are no whole grain options for things such as croissants, doughnuts, and white cake. The very idea of a whole grain doughnut makes me laugh, since there is no way it can be the same as those airy things with the chocolate frosting. But there must be another food that would satisfy you instead. What about warm brown rice topped with butter, whole wheat bread spread with peanut butter, oatmeal Apple Pancakes (recipe in Chapter 11), a latte (remember, this means a latte without caramel or special sweeteners). Go on a hunt for comfort foods with your friends and see how many different ones you can come up with. You may find alternatives that work just as well as your old favorites. Our friends on the website have this discussion every few months. It's a hot topic for all of us. Food as comfort is high on the list.

Think about what kinds of foods might comfort you so you can make them when you need them. Start by identifying the specific characteristic of your comfort food that is comforting. Does your comfort food need to be warm? Does it need to be soft in your mouth? Here are some things that our readers have reported using as comfort foods instead of white things. Recipes for foods with asterisks are in Chapter 11.

- Italian Frittata*
- Crustless Quiche*
- Quesadillas on whole wheat or corn tortilla
- Burrito on whole wheat tortilla
- Pizza with Whole Wheat Crust
- Cornbread
- Oatmeal Muffins*
- Cottage Cheese–Cinnamon Pancakes*
- Tomato soup made with milk and topped with basil and a pat of butter
- Split pea soup (add turkey sausage or bacon bits)
- Cream of chicken soup with extra chicken added
- Oven-Fried Sweet Potatoes*
- Sweet Potato Pie*
- Oatmeal-Apple Pancakes
- Ricotta-Fruit "Pudding"*
- Chili Layered Casserole*

Also take a look at the dessert recipes in Chapter 11.

Figure out your list and then make sure you buy what you need when you go to the grocery store. If your comfort food is in your cupboard or refrigerator when you want it, you are less likely to go on a prowl and find the real thing.

Desserts That Work for You

Yes, you can keep your commitment to brown things and still eat dessert. Did you notice the desserts suggested in the section above on elegant dinners? There are dessert recipes in Chapter 11, too. They include Squash Pie, Carrot Cake, Pumpkin Tofu Cheesecake, and Pumpkin Cake with Cashew Butter Frosting. It is important that you sort out whether or not you will be okay with desserts. Some people take great comfort in brown desserts, find them a useful addition to their plan, and like making them. Others have found that dessert of any kind reminds them of the old days of sugar-laden foods. They are a major trigger food for them. Even healthy dessert alternatives serve as a trigger—just thinking about dessert makes them want more, and more of the real thing. Your job is to sort out what is right for you.

Tips from the Field: Try This Treat

Sometimes for dessert I will have fried bananas. Melt some butter in a nonstick frying pan, add walnuts and cinnamon, and cook until nuts are toasty. Then break a green banana into chunks and add it to the pan. Cook until it is nicely yellowed and coated with the cinnamon butter.

—C.

8

Taking the Sugars Out:
Step 6

You may feel ambivalent about the next step of your program—taking the sugars out. You may swing between dreading giving up sugars and barely keeping yourself from leaping ahead and chucking everything. Or you may have ignored my earlier advice totally: ditched all sugars the second day of your program, felt horrible, and started over again. But either way, we have now come to Step 6.

If you've been doing the steps in order, going off sugars is the logical next step. You may find it isn't all that dramatic. It will be just one more adjustment to your carbohydrates so that you eat as few simple carbohydrates (sugars and white things) as possible. And you will be making that change in the context of being consistent with your three meals a day with protein, your nightly spud, your food journal, your browns vs. whites.

Being stable is the first of the three keys to success with this step. The second is understanding the big picture about you and sweet foods. You may have already started to see this by studying your food journal and looking at the relationship between your feelings and the foods you eat and identifying any addictive relationships you have with sweet and white foods.

In the next three chapters, we will work on practical ways to take sugar out of your diet and heal your emotional cravings for food as love. You will learn a mental exercise called reframing. Rather than associating eating milk and cookies with love, you will consciously start noticing other alternatives, not associated with food, that are better for your body. Sugar as love will no longer be the marker and measure of your life. When you start this process, this idea may seem pretty far-fetched, but I promise that over time, it will begin to make more sense.

Having the plan work for you in this phase will require paying attention in a deeper way. You will learn to recognize those foods that can set you off. You will learn to spot a food with covert sugar in it a mile away. This phase of your food plan will teach you to read labels, recognize sugar's many aliases, and choose to eat foods that are not filled with sugars. Step 6 has two parts. The first involves going off what I call overt sugars—the candy, cake, pie, soda, and cookies that you love so much. The second involves taking out the covert sugar—the sugars like high-fructose corn syrup hidden in other foods. You can choose to do both at once or to ease into it by doing the overt sugars first and then tackling the covert sugars.

By now, you eat whatever sugars you are still having with your meals. Your sugar binges are probably a great deal less intense. You may have found that you have already significantly and naturally reduced your sugar intake. As you know, sugar affects you like a drug. If you think of going off sugars as a drug detoxification process, you can help your mind and body minimize the discomfort of the transition. You can keep the detox in perspective. Your beta-endorphin receptors will not be happy about your taking sugars out. They will tell you in no uncertain terms by creating headaches, irritability, and edginess. I will guide you through the sugar detox process and help you teach your beta-endorphin receptors to quiet down and adjust to your new sugar-free life.

Let's take a look at the three parts to a successful long-term sugar detox:

1. Be really consistent with the earlier steps of the plan: The stronger the foundation, the easier going off sugar will be. If you have taken a sufficient amount of time to allow your body to adjust to the changes you are making, your sugar detox will not be difficult. If you rush things, you can get into difficulty. I generally encourage people to spend at least eight to ten weeks getting solid with the program before they consider a sugar detox.

2. Understand the emotional cues (like love) that you associate with certain foods. For many people, especially women, sugar foods are strongly connected to feeling safe and loved. Your detox may evoke feelings of abandonment and sadness. You may feel as if you are giving up your best friend. Do not dismiss or make light of these feelings. If you don't honor them, they will sabotage your commitment to be sugar-free.

3. Keep an eye on the details of how much sugar is in the foods you eat. Sugars are hidden everywhere. Once you have shifted to a sugar-free state, your body will be far more sensitive to the drug effect of sugars. If the foods you eat are loaded with covert sugar, you can activate your craving for sugar without intending to. You will need to protect yourself from using sugars when you don't want to.

Tips from the Field: Time to Go Back to Basics?

As I work with the program, I continue to get new revelations. First of all, it took me a while to realize that one step at a time means one step at a time. After several setbacks, I realized that I had never really gotten the three meals a day down before I moved on. Looking back at the steps, it suddenly hit me in the face: "It won't work if you don't do the steps."

—P.

Setting the Stage

Let's make sure you are ready for this next phase of your program. There are several ways to go off sugars:

1. Slowly decrease the amount of sugars you use until you no longer wish to have any.
2. Go off overt sugars all at once and then gradually decrease the amount of covert sugars you use.
3. Go off all sugars all at once.

Which of these three you choose will depend upon your own style. The second method seems to be the easiest approach for most people. The actual sugar withdrawal or detox from overt sugars takes about five days. If you are not using huge amounts of covert sugars at the same time, it is a reasonable and manageable transition. As you may have already learned, if you are using a great deal of sugar and stop abruptly, you will be miserable.

But whichever way you choose, we want to ensure that the stability you have created up to this point will hold you through your sugar detox. Your first task includes a little housecleaning— both physical (in your kitchen) and emotional (with your family and friends). Let's start with the easier one.

Cleaning Your Kitchen

Go into your kitchen, open your cabinets, and take out all the foods with obvious sugars in them. This includes leftover Halloween or other candy, high-sugar comfort foods, soda, sugary cereals such as Frosted Flakes—you know, all the high-temptation stuff. Throw it away or give it away. Ideally, see if you can get every last bit of it out of the house.

If your family will go nuts if you give away their sugar foods, arrange with them to put all the sweet things into one place. Choose a cupboard or cabinet that you do not usually use. Call it the sugar stash. You will know what is there, but at least you can make the choice whether to go and look at or eat what is in the cupboard. By separating the sugar stash from the other foods, you will at least minimize your bumping into such foods while you are trying to be "clean."

Talking to Your Family and Friends

The next step is an emotional housecleaning. So far, your family and friends have probably seen the positive change in you as you progress with this program. They may have seen that overall you have more energy, are more upbeat, relaxed, and sympathetic. They know you aren't "fixed" yet, but they are interested in the change that is taking place in you. Some family members may have rolled their eyes at first when they heard you were on another diet, but they have probably changed their tune by now.

But now that you are going to stop eating sugar, their reactions may well change again. They may be worried that you are going to expect them to stop eating sugar, too. They may be fiercely resistant or totally uninterested in anything that has to do with your eating more regularly and giving up sugar. They may even actively subvert your commitment to the plan. Your husband may ask, "Are you still doing that stuff?" as he orders chocolate mousse for dessert. Your kids may unconsciously try to sabotage you as well. Remember, sugar sensitivity is inherited. The chances that your family is sugar sensitive are really high. You know this. They know this. And they may not be in the same place you are, ready to move toward a sugar-free life.

You may also have close friends who are sugar sensitive. And friends who are still very attached to sugar and white things may warn you of the dangers of a "high-protein diet." Telling them that this food plan is not a high-protein diet will have no impact, because the concern isn't really about protein. They are worried that if you change, they may feel pressured to change as well. And many people are not ready to. You can't clear out your husband or unsupportive best friend the way you can clear out your cabinet, but you can be clear with them and clear in your own mind and commitment. And you can actively add other people to your support group.

You need support from people who understand your program. Talking with folks who are supportive is absolutely critical to your success. You could do this by doing the program with a friend, joining a local Potatoes Not Prozac support group, or finding a way to get online and talk to the great folks on the website. However you choose to find support, make a real effort to do so! It will make a world of difference to the success of your program. Having a personal connection to others doing the program will help you stick with it.

Tips from the Field:
The Drawbacks of a Husband Who Cooks

When I started on your plan, I was reminded of Al-Anon, which tries to help families understand the changes that their newly sober spouse/parent is going through. The difference is that "I've lost my drinking companion" translates to "It's no fun to eat ice cream unless you do."

For example, my husband loves to prepare meals, but I have to spoil some of his menu plans. This morning he was looking forward to us having a rich coffee cake he had bought, and I had to beg off. He's trying to be very cooperative, but just doesn't understand yet. I guess the secret is to ease the family into change.

—A.

Having Second Thoughts

As you start getting ready for your sugar detox, you may have second thoughts about whether you really want to do this. Feelings of sadness may emerge. You may wonder if you really want a sugar-free life. You may feel really sad that you will never have sweet things again. Sweet foods are so much a part of celebrations, of holidays, of family togetherness. How will you manage this?

This is a natural feeling. All of us know it well. Usually it is far more intense at the very beginning of doing the program than at this stage, because in later steps you already have had the experience of feeling so much better thanks to the program. Your brain and body know this is the right plan for you. But the feelings of loss may remain. This loss is real and valid. Our culture uses sugar to celebrate special events, to show love, and to provide comfort, so it can be difficult staying sugar-free in such an environment.

But alternatives do exist. Making special Christmas tree ornaments can take the place of baking and icing Christmas cookies; giving flowers can replace giving candy; soup and an offer of comfort can be given instead of bread. Your old "food as love" associations will change over time. Just be gentle with yourself.

Holding the Sadness

A key part of getting ready to take the sugars out is acknowledging the intensity of the emotional cues associated with sugars in our culture. Many of your childhood memories of support and love are connected to food, usually sweet or white foods. They hold a very big emotional charge for you.

But the foods you think of as providing comfort are the very things that have contributed to your problems. In other words, oftentimes the reason you *need* comfort is due to the very sweet or white food you are eating!

This is a very difficult concept to explain to someone who is still using comfort foods. When you are caught in the middle of these foods, it is almost impossible to understand how big a problem they are creating.

An alcoholic who is still drinking will often tell me, "I would stop drinking if I could just get my life squared away." And she will struggle and struggle and struggle to fix her problems, but they still surround her and create her need for a drink. Using sugars and white things acts in exactly the same way. I used to feel I needed a hot fudge sundae every night after work because my work was so stressful, so demanding, and so tiring. I had no idea that it was the hot fudge sundae that was significantly contributing to the stress of my life. My sugar-laden brain could not in any way make that connection.

Because you have been doing the plan for a while now, I know this concept is starting to make sense to you. You can see more clearly the huge effect that these sugar foods have on you. You recognize that your down sides are directly correlated to what you are eating. So on an intellectual level you are ready. On an emotional level, though, you may continue to be scared about having to give things up that have so much tenderness associated with them.

After all is said and done, ultimately you will be making a choice about what you want more. I still miss those green-iced Christmas cookies. I still want them every Christmas. Time has not made it easier. But experience has. I want my recovery more than I want the *illusion* of comfort that those cookies would give me. You will grow into this place, too. The longer you do the program, the more this will make sense to you.

Planning for the Big Day

Detoxing from sugar will call upon you to use all your knowledge about giving your body the right foods at the right times to keep your sugar-sensitive brain chemistry balanced. More than ever, you will need to eat regular meals with protein, and you will need to do so with consistency, day after day, week after week. This is where the stability you established earlier in the program really pays off.

When you decide you are ready for a full detox, remember that it will take five days and you may experience some withdrawal symptoms. If you get really uncomfortable during this time, have an apple with some protein as a snack. But take care not to start eating a whole lot of fruit. Fruit contains a sugar called fructose. Different fruits have a different sugar impact. The intensity of the effect is related to the amount of fiber in the fruit. Strawberries, raspberries, and blueberries will affect you far less than mangoes and papaya. If you have fruit, have it with protein. Eat fruits with skin and slow down the sugar effect. More fiber gives you a slower sugar effect. Some fruit may work for you, but it may trigger cravings. Be attentive, use your journal, and as always, ask your body what is best.

This is one of the many new ways in which you will need to pay attention to the details of what you eat and the effect it has on your mood and your body. Some people, for example, are triggered by the sugar found naturally in milk (lactose). Others (like me) get triggered by whole wheat pasta, but have no trouble eating brown rice pasta. You will have to discover for yourself what your trigger foods are. Let your food journal help you do this. Continue to record your food and your feelings, and when you think you have spotted a trigger food, look further back in your journal to see what effects that food had on you earlier in the program.

Rigorous vs. Flexible

When you were just starting on your program, it worked better to ease into sugar awareness and cut down if you were able. As you move into the detox phase of your recovery, you will want to be more attentive to sugars in their many forms. How much covert sugar you will use will be determined by listening to your body. If you eat a certain food during detox and you find yourself wanting more of it, planning to go to the store and buy it, keeping a stash of it in the house, thinking of new ways to cook it, it is probably a food you should avoid! Read the label and make a choice.

Some people ask me, "How many grams of sugar *can* I have?" If you have a number, then you will continue to calculate grams rather than working with your body. There is no absolute value to use as a guide. The more you can connect with the idea of being a sugar addict, the easier this process will be. But ultimately, your recovery is about your being in relationship to what your body is telling you. You can now discern what is right for you.

Be sure to note all your reactions to food in your journal. And don't just write down the feelings you have at the moment you are eating. Write down your feelings whenever you notice them. If you don't happen to have your journal with you, write down what you are feeling on any piece of paper that's at hand. Include the date and time. Then you can transfer this information into your food journal when you have time.

Spotting Sugars

Overt Sugars

Whether you have decided to do your detox slowly or all at once, you need to know your sugars. Overt sugars are the ones that look like sugar. You may have classified some overt sugars as healthy ones. For example, you may have thought that honey was better for you than white sugar because it comes from a natural source. Your sugar-sensitive body does not make this distinction. Whether the sugar is natural or refined, your reaction will be the same. And the more intense the sugar, the more intense your reaction.

Here are the sugars usually classified as overt:

White sugar	Honey
Brown sugar	Molasses
Powdered sugar	Maple syrup
Turbinado or	Corn syrup (also known as high-
raw sugar	fructose corn syrup)

The hard-line sweet foods you all know so well are the ones that are high in overt sugars. These include Coke, ice cream, doughnuts, candy bars, cake, pie, cookies, etc. I have never met a sugar-sensitive person who was not an expert on overt sugar foods.

Covert Sugars

Covert sugars are those that are hidden in processed foods. They can be highly concentrated and make up a large part of a food or they can be a small amount added for "taste." They range from the high-fructose corn syrup found in many processed foods to the hidden sugar in canned vegetables or ketchup. It sometimes requires a little detective work to find them. Read food labels and learn to identify foods where covert sugars are hiding.

You will find that many packaged foods also have covert sugars in them. Check the labels of things like Carnation Instant Breakfast, tomato soup, bran muffins, barbecue sauce, Power Bars, fruit drinks, and even frozen dinners. Check your box of salt. You will be floored to discover where our covert friends appear. Sugar is everywhere.

The sugars listed below are some of the sugars that wait in processed foods to ambush your recovery. The sugar industry has creative chemists. Sugar sells.

Some marketing ads will make claims that a certain product made with sugars has a low glycemic impact. These sugars may affect your blood sugar/insulin response differently. But the sweet taste evokes beta-endorphin, which primes you to want more and more sugar. Even a sugar that is lower in its glycemic response may have a huge priming effect on your sugar-sensitive brain. Be attentive to labels. And, even more important, be attentive to your body. If you find yourself feeling crabby and out of sorts, go back to your journal, see what you ate, and then go read the label. If you are craving sweets or white things, you have been primed. Something has sneaked in and activated your sugar-sensitive system. Pay attention if you are craving or noticing sweet things. You may discover one of these covert sugar products in the foods you have eaten:

Amasake	Dextrose
Apple sugar	Diglycerides
Barbados sugar	Disaccharides
Bark sugar	Evaporated cane juice
(Zylose)	Florida crystals
Barley malt	Fructooligosaccharides (FOS)
Barley malt syrup	Fructose
Beet sugar	Fruit juice concentrate
Brown rice syrup	Galactose
Cane juice	Glucose
Cane sugar	Glucitol
Cane syrup	Glucoamine
Carbitol	Gluconolactone (may be found
Caramel coloring	in tofu)
Caramel sugars	Glucose
Caramelized foods	Glucose polymers
Concentrated fruit juice	Glucose syrup
Corn sweetener	Glycerides
D-tagalose	Glycerine
Date sugar	Glycerol
Dextrin	Glycol

High-fructose corn syrup

Inversol

Invert sugar

Isomalt

Karo syrups

Lactose

Levulose

"Lite" sugar

"Light" sugar

Malt dextrin

Malted barley

Maltose

Maltodextrins

Maltodextrose

Malts (any)

Mannitol, sorbitol, xylitol, maltitol

Mannose

Microcrystalline cellulose

Molasses

Monoglycerides

Monosaccharides

Nectars

Neotame

Pentose

Polydextrose

Polyglycerides

Raisin juice

Raisin syrup

Ribose rice syrup

Rice malt

Rice sugar

Rice sweeteners

Rice syrup solids

Saccharides (any)

Sorbitol (aka Hexitol)

Sorghum

Sucanat (evaporated cane juice)

Sucanet

Sucrose

Sugar cane

Trisaccharides

Unrefined sugar

Zylos

It is also important to understand how food labels work. Legally, if the chemical structure of a carbohydrate has more than two sugar molecules, it will be called a complex carbohydrate on a food label instead of a sugar. So the label may show that a certain food has no sugar and 35 grams of carbohydrate. But if that carbohydrate is maltodextrin, your sugar-sensitive body will respond to it as a sugar. Read the food labels in detail, and pay attention to the ingredient list rather than the grams of sugar listed to learn the subtleties of where sugars are hidden.

Low-fat products often hide a lot of sugar. When food manufacturers take out the fat, sugars are used to enhance taste. Also, take a close look at foods that proclaim "no sugar." Remember that in the land of food labeling, "no sugar" simply means "no sucrose." Food manufacturers use different kinds of sweeteners to mask how much sugar is in products marketed as "healthy" or "low fat." The labels on these foods may show five different ingredients, such as malt dextrin, raisin juice, or fructose. These all sound healthy, don't they? They are all sugars. Your taste buds and your addictive body chemistry will recognize them as sugars even though the label may say "sugar free." Read labels carefully.

Pay attention to where sugar is hidden in restaurant foods as well. Chinese food and Thai food, for example, are both very high in sugar. If you have gone through a sugar detox and then go out for a nice "healthy" stir-fry with shrimp and bok choy, you may find yourself with inexplicable cravings the next morning. There was sugar in the stir-fry sauce. I have had this experience even after asking the Chinese restaurant to prepare my food without sugar. You'll find more information on dining out in Chapter 10.

Artificial Sweeteners

I do not encourage your using artificial sweeteners as an alternative to sugars for a number of reasons. The *taste* of sweet, whether from table sugar, corn syrup, or aspartame, evokes a beta-endorphin response in your body. This reaction will create cravings. Essentially, artificial sweeteners, while not evoking the same insulin response, will prime your brain to want more "sweet." This sets you up to go back to the sugars.

In addition, most sugar-free products use aspartame (Nutra-sweet) as a sweetener. Aspartame is made from phenylala-nine, which is an amino acid. Having a lot of phenylalanine can be a problem for a number of reasons. It is a precursor to dopamine (the same way that tryptophan is a precursor for serotonin). Dopamine is the neurotransmitter that creates a feeling of brightness and excitement in your brain. You like the dopamine effects in your brain. They are considered potent reinforcers. Dopamine is the neurotransmitter affected by cocaine.

I have observed that a very large number of sugar addicts are dependent upon sugar-free products. My hypothesis is that the phenylalanine evokes dopamine and creates an upper-like effect. I suspect that sugar-sensitive people get a bigger reaction to this than do people who are not. This drug effect can be addictive, sometimes as addictive as sugar. Caffeine in diet sodas heightens the effect even more.

Do not switch to sugar-free products as a way to ease into a sugar-free life. If you are already strongly attached to them, work on holding your "dose" steady while you detox from regular sugars. You can then work on a sugar-free detox down the line. I do not recommend going off sugar-free products all at once. Cut down over time and use your journal to guide your progress.

Being Attentive to Your Plan

Detoxing from sugar will call upon you to use all your skills and knowledge about giving your body the right foods at the right times to keep your sugar-sensitive brain chemistry balanced. In the detox phase, more than ever, you will need to eat regular meals with protein, and you will need to do so consistently, day after day, week after week. This is where the stability you established earlier in the program really pays off. Pay close attention to your food journal. And to make your detox easier, increase your vegetables a lot *before* you start it.

Here's why. Vegetables are carbohydrates. They are actually very slo-o-o-o-o-w sugars. They will give your body a sense of being satisfied without cravings. They will not prime you to want

more and go on a quest—no one goes out to the convenience
store in the middle of the night to find some frozen peas!

Also pay attention to your vitamins and the other supports
(water and exercise) to your program.

Let's just check in on your vitamin plan:

- **Vitamin C.** 500 to 5,000 mg a day, depending on what
  your system needs. Doctors skilled in vitamin C
  supplementation often suggest a "bowel tolerance"
  dosage. That means starting low and adding a little more
  vitamin C each day. If you find yourself having gas,
  diarrhea, or stomach distress, cut your dosage back by
  500 mg at a time until the symptoms subside. You may
  find that the lower dosage works just fine for you unless
  you are getting sick. Then increasing the dosage would
  be warranted.
- **Vitamin B complex.** 50 mg a day. You can take the
  B-complex in either tablet or liquid form. I prefer the
  liquid because it allows you to take a smaller amount several
  times a day. This reduces the likelihood of stomach upset.
  Do not take B-complex at night, because it may keep you up.
- **Zinc.** 15 mg a day.

Why these three vitamins for your plan? Vitamin C, a B-complex
vitamin, and zinc are traditionally used in alcohol detox. Since
sugar addiction is so closely linked to the metabolic pathways of
alcoholism, this triple package can work wonders for your healing process.

Vitamin C is the busiest of the plan vitamins. It:

- Speeds detoxification by acting as a scavenger that
  consumes free radicals (by-products of toxin activity
  within your body).

- Helps your adrenals recover from adrenal fatigue coming from stress and the high levels of sugar.
- Helps convert the amino acid tryptophan (found in the protein you eat) into serotonin.

The B vitamins are essential in breaking down carbohydrates so the body can burn them as fuel. One of the B vitamins, niacin, is critical to the conversion of tryptophan into serotonin. B vitamins affect many functions in your body. Each B vitamin does a slightly different task. They work best when in balance and working together. Some people attempt to choose a particular B vitamin to maximize the given effect. I encourage you not to split them up. Take a complex of B vitamins. It will work better in your body.

Zinc affects a wide variety of functions in your body. The most intriguing are its effects on glucose tolerance and insulin sensitivity. Adequate levels of zinc make a huge difference in how your body utilizes glucose. Good zinc, good absorption. If the sugar in your blood is actually used and burned, it is less likely to be stored as fat in your body.

Don't Forget the Water and Exercise

Sometimes as people get further along in their program, they backslide a bit on some of the basics like water and exercise.

Drink eight to ten glasses of water each day. (If you weigh more than 200 pounds, drink more than that. Use a rough guideline of drinking half your body weight in ounces of water per day.) If you have drifted away from drinking enough water, get started again! It will be even more crucial as you start your sugar detox.

I find it hard to fill up my water glass and drink it down eight times a day. But I can fill my 32-ounce plastic water bottle a couple of times and simply sip from it throughout my day. Find whatever works for you and do it.

I am often asked to suggest alternatives to drinking soda. I say, "Drink water." "But, Kathleen, water is boring," people reply. And I say, "Yup, water is boring." But that boring old water will help to heal your sugar addiction. Drink water. Add a slice of lemon if it makes water more interesting to you. Try different herbal teas. Discover the difference in flavor of the mint teas.

Exercise is particularly helpful during detox. Sugar-sensitive people seem to either not exercise at all or exercise compulsively. While I certainly do not expect that you will remake your entire exercise program before doing your detox, being consistent about it will help in going off sugars.

At the very least, get out and walk every day for twenty minutes. Ten minutes out, ten minutes in. And if you can get to the gym and do a little workout, that will be even better. Cranking up your exercise enhances every part of your body and your program.

Tips from the Field: Call It "Movement"

I work with a personal trainer once per week, as this is very motivating for me. One thing she has really helped me with is substituting the word "movement" for the word "exercise." Any movement is exercise! What a liberating thing! If I get up and change the TV channel vs. using the remote, that's exercise! If I take the stairs instead of the elevator, that's exercise. If I talk on the cordless phone and walk around dusting while I'm talking, that's exercise. It is amazing how much movement can change our lives, no matter what our size. (I am overweight by 100 pounds—and on my way down!) I do a lot of water aerobics, because we weigh only 10 percent of our weight in water (yippee) so there's a lot less stress on our joints.

—L.

The Sugar/Alcohol Dilemma

A number of sugar-sensitive people use alcohol to relax and deal with stress. Some of you may be dependent upon alcohol. Since alcohol is a sugar, going off alcohol will be part of your sugar detox. If you are alcohol dependent, you will be going off of alcohol as a part of your sugar detox. If alcohol is part of your sugar addiction, you will need to do some extra planning.

Oftentimes people will ask me how they can know if they have a problem with alcohol. In a clinical setting, we can assess whether you have a problem with alcohol, and if you do, determine the severity of the problem. If you don't have access to that kind of evaluation, you may be having a few drinks before dinner or wine with dinner and not know if it is a problem.

The simplest way to find out is to try to stop. If you find that you want to stop but find it difficult, you have a problem. If you can stop but are spending a huge amount of energy in managing not to have a drink, you have a problem.

You may not like the simplicity and definitive part of these assessments. You may want to argue with me, but I think of alcohol dependence as simply an extension of sugar sensitivity. If you are highly sensitive to sugars, you will be even more sensitive to alcohol.

If you find yourself trying to convince yourself (or me in your mind) that the few drinks before dinner can't possibly mean you have a problem, that is one more clue. People who do not have a problem with alcohol simply stop having it. They do not argue or cut deals or manage their use of it.

Staying Safe

If alcohol is part of your sugar addiction, it will be important for you to adapt your detox plan. Do an alcohol detox *before* you do your entire sugar detox. If you are having more than three drinks a day, seek professional support in going off alcohol. Do not think you can do this alone. Find support in your community. Find another person who is in recovery from alcohol addiction and who understands what you are going through. If you cannot find a person who understands sugar addiction and alcohol dependence, come to the website at www.radiantrecovery.com.

Final Preparations

Picking a Time

Now you are ready to go for it. You have done your homework and know the drill. When you detox from sugar, you will go through something similar to a drug detox, but it will be less extreme. Because your sugar-sensitive body reacts to sugar as if it were a drug, you may have withdrawal symptoms. Your brain will be begging you to eat some sugar. You may get the shakes, feel nauseous and edgy, or have diarrhea or headaches for a few days. That's normal—and it's why you need to plan your sugar detox for a time when you will not be under severe stress. But remember, if you have been doing the steps in the recovery program for a while, these symptoms will be far less severe than if you simply were to go cold turkey on day one.

The actual sugar detox process usually takes five days, with the fourth day being the hardest. You will want to really *plan* the timing of your detox. Schedule it so that on the fourth day you have time to yourself. Give yourself space so you can be cranky or have the physical withdrawal symptoms without their affecting your big meeting at work or your daughter's wedding day.

Be strategic about this and you'll be successful. Chances are, you'll wake up on the fifth morning of your detox feeling great!

Knowing Your Style

Getting ready for your detox should include a review of your style of making change. Let's take a look at a few helpful questions.

When you have to do something, do you like to get all your ducks in a row, then work through each task one at a time? Or do you like to jump in and start doing it all at once? Now ask yourself the same question about your sugar detox. Are you going to ease into it or are you going to just *do* it? Are you going to cut down slowly or cut out all sugar at once?

Do this step in whatever style you like to do other things in your life. Over the years, most of my clients have used a combination of approaches. They cut down on white things and sugars first, then pick a time to go cold turkey and eliminate whatever sugars are left in their diets. This seems to work best for most people, but again, *do what's right for you.* If the detox style fits your natural rhythm, it is more likely to work smoothly and successfully.

No Sugars!

Pick your day. This is the start of no sugars. Read labels, be vigilant. Choose the degree of attentiveness you will have in your own detox.

When you are doing a detox, however, being strict with yourself seems to work better at the beginning. While the actual biochemical detox will take five days or so, the emotional detachment may take a few months. I find that it is easier to decide not to have any sugars than to constantly slip around trying to figure out how much is right. But if you feel that being totally strict will not work for you, listen to yourself and create your own way. The most important instruction here is to feel comfortable with what you can do. This is *your* healing plan for *your* body.

There's one thing you do want to be aware of, though. Denial is a powerful operating factor in addiction. Sometimes, in the name of being kind to oneself, sugar-sensitive people will be slow or sloppy about actually getting off sugars. So pay close attention to your process. Ask yourself your motivation in designing your plan. Are you going slowly because it's healthy or because you don't want to let go of your best friend? Be honest. The results you will get are well worth the work you will do on this one.

Tips from the Field: Take as Much Time as You Need

Remember to keep in mind that this program is a PROCESS . . . a JOURNEY. Take it slow and be gentle with yourself along the way. I'm preaching to myself here, too, believe me. I love Frappuccinos. They are a major hit of caffeine and sugar! I used to have a Frappuccino every day. I'm now down to one per week, and this is major progress for me. I have to look at how far I've come, and not allow myself to dwell on how far I have to go.

I think when I am ready to completely give up Frappuccinos, it will not be a traumatic event. Even now, they are losing their hold on me. I can drive by a coffee shop without stopping. I don't even gaze longingly in the windows. I can visualize life without Frappuccinos. I know it's coming!

—*L.*

I never believed I could get off sugar. But understanding that the feelings were withdrawal helped a lot. I made it through three days and was ready to quit. The fourth day was horrible. I felt like I wanted to bite my boss's head off. I went home early and just kept eating those three meals with protein. Mr. Spud helped, too. On the fifth day, I woke up and felt clear and peaceful. I couldn't believe it! It keeps getting better. Is this magic or what?

—*K.*

What to Eat

Let's take a look at how you can support your detox even more. What you eat in this phase makes a big difference in how successful you will be. By now you are eating plenty of protein three times a day and have gotten yourself pretty much shifted from white things to brown things. You are being diligent about Mr. Spud every night and are taking your vitamins every day. In many cases, this shift will have already eliminated a fair amount of the sugar in your diet.

Before you take the plunge and drop more things out of your food plan, let's add something. Make sure that you are getting regular browns in each meal. Having a sufficient amount of complex carbohydrates will substantially decrease the discomfort of your detox. Have whole grain bread, brown rice, potatoes with skins, beans, oatmeal, nuts, whole wheat pasta, and the like.

Eating more veggies, especially dense ones like broccoli and cauliflower (I know, I know, it seems really weird to talk about cauliflower when you are trying to pay attention to sugar), will help the transition. Butternut squash with nutmeg and cheese can ease a whole lot of sugar sadness.

So now you have a solid food plan, are emotionally stable, and are doing the vitamins, the spud, and the veggies. You are ready. Let's do it!

Your Actual Detox

After all this preparation, your actual detox will go pretty smoothly. After many years of hearing how people go through this process, I am amazed at how direct and simple it is. In many ways it is kind of anticlimactic. Sugar detox has the biggest negative charge when you try to do it as Step 1. Then it makes you off the wall, nasty, not at all pleasant to be around. Then you could only go three days before giving in and eating sugar again.

But when you do your detox after all the work on the first five steps, it will seem natural, logical, and not at all difficult. And best of all, you will have a huge sense of satisfaction. You will be doing what you have tried to do a thousand times before. But this time it will work!

The Big Day!

Pick your no-sugar day carefully. Choose a time when you will have five days without a major event. You have cleaned your cupboards. You have warned your family. Be especially vigilant about your food during this time, take your vitamins, and make sure to have Mr. Spud nightly. Keep busy. If you are cranky or edgy, go for a walk. Go to the gym. Swim, lift weights, and sit in the hot tub. Go to a museum; take your kids to the zoo. Don't go to a movie; you will want popcorn and a candy bar. The entire movie environment is designed to get you to eat. Stay away from dangerous places for the time being.

Stay busy so you don't get bored and want to eat as a way to cope. Get connected to your support network. Write in your journal. Sing, dance, laugh, make love ... even if you are crabby. These things help raise your beta-endorphin levels.

Here are a few other ideas from folks in the Community Forum:

- *I take a bubble bath, maybe even by candlelight.*
- *I just sit outside when I am not up to really doing anything. I might take a book or something, but mostly I just soak in the out-of-doors, the light, the breeze, the sights.*
- *I like to listen to a comforting CD.*
- *I feel a lot better just by bringing fresh flowers into my home.*
- *I curl up and watch the old Jimmy Stewart movie* It's a Wonderful Life.
- *My cure for crabbiness is to put lavender essential oil on my pillow and down comforter, and take an afternoon nap.*

Most important, don't spook yourself. Doing a sugar detox does *not* have to be a big thing. It is only that way if you do it off the bat without a safety net. But you are ready, you are informed, and you have been practicing. Think of this as simply one more step on your path. I know you can do it!

Tips from the Field: One Meal at a Time

The best advice I ever got about this program is this: Just keep making the best meal choice you can—one meal at a time.

—*M.*

Life After Detox

Your sugar detox is not the end of the addiction story; it is the beginning of a new way of living. You will start to adjust to a sugar-free life. You may be very excited and diligent for months. At some point, sugar will call you. Doughnuts will hop into your mouth unexpectedly, someone will bring a box of your favorite chocolates, or Girl Scout cookie time will arrive; you will forget your resolve and have some sugar. Because your brain has now adapted to life without sugar, the first taste and response to the sugar will be wonderful. You will feel euphoric, mellow, and very comforted. Your addictive brain will tell you that just a little bit is all right. Your addictive brain is very seductive and *loves* the feelings that come with sugar. It will try to make you forget the old days of addiction and seduce you into thinking that you are healed and can now have some sugar in moderation.

During the time you were sugar free, your beta-endorphin receptors have upregulated. You now have more of them. The more rigorous you have been, the more sites you have grown. When you have sugar, you activate all the new ones. When they empty out, they will scream big-time. They will object more than they did before. Your craving will wake up and insist, demand, and cry for more sweet stuff. Your addictive brain will tell you that you can manage it. It will say that just a little will be okay. More than likely, you will slip into a wobbly place.

The wobbly place is a critical juncture for you. If you are attentive and remember the seductive nature of your addictive brain, you will forgive yourself the little slip and go back to your regular recovery plan. Three meals with protein, brown foods, and Mr. Spud. You will be kind to the screaming beta-endorphin sites, eat an apple with cheese, and give away the Girl Scout cookies.

And if by chance your wobble becomes a full-blown relapse, you will be kind to yourself and remember that all of us have been there. Healing from addiction means coming back from relapse. You don't have to feel guilty or beat yourself up; just come home to the program and start again. Think of it as a learning experience and come home to recovery.

Holding true to a life of recovery over the long haul is a process. You don't get there straight off. You get better and better after each slip or relapse. You learn to get more support, you get stronger in your commitment, you become more attached to feeling good. And somewhere down the line, your love of recovery is so strong that nothing will get in the way of it. Chocolate won't be worth it. Girl Scout cookies will make you smile. You will feel filled up rather than deprived. And you won't trade the feelings for anything.

9

Staying with the Program over Time: Step 7

Working your program over time takes some practice. There are a set of skills that will help you get through the transition to an easy sugar-free life. Let's take a look at some of them that will help you with Step 7: Create a new life.

Socializing Without Sugars

So many social gatherings—from holiday dinners to tailgate parties or Fourth of July picnics—revolve around food, usually foods that are not the best for you: grilled hot dogs and hamburgers on fluffy white buns, mashed potatoes and biscuits, strawberry shortcake, apple pie. But you can stick with your plan even at special events. Let me suggest a new way of planning for these times and creating alternatives for special occasions.

Christmas is the granddaddy of all sugar holidays. If you celebrate Christmas or just work in an office and are a sugar addict, you will struggle with wanting to eat sweets around the holidays. But there are creative solutions. You might take heart and inspiration from Gretel, who brainstormed on the forum about how she reframed her usual associations with Christmas. This is her list:

- Christmas is *The Nutcracker Suite* with sugar plum fairies.
- Christmas is Hansel and Gretel and gingerbread houses.
- Christmas is roasting chestnuts (or marshmallows) on an open fire.
- Christmas is eggnog.
- Christmas is leaving milk and cookies for Santa.
- Christmas is stockings filled with candy, fruit, and nuts.
- Christmas is Christmas cookies.
- Christmas is baking cakes, pies, and breads to share.
- Christmas is caroling and stopping for hot chocolate afterward.
- Christmas is open houses with food and drink I don't have control over.
- Christmas is office parties I don't plan.

Then she asked herself what Christmas *might* mean if she took all the Christmas foods out of the equation and looked at the bigger picture. She decided to include her spiritual self. Here's what she discovered:

- Christmas is the birth of a child.
- Christmas is giving.
- Christmas is celebration.
- Christmas is beautiful music.
- Christmas is twinkling lights on a starlit night.
- Christmas is snow glistening in the sunlight.
- Christmas is Santa coming down the chimney.
- Christmas is puppies and kittens.
- Christmas is surprises.
- Christmas is love.

- Christmas is family.
- Christmas is friends.

Gretel reframed her old associations of food with love. Socializing without sugar is not that difficult if you can shift your energy to the *meaning* of the holiday or special occasion rather than the food.

If sweets are given to you at the office or at your place of work, give them to your non-sugar-sensitive friends. You can reframe any holiday in this same way. Simply focus on non-food things as an expression of your love. Enlist your friends and families in this process. They may be dismayed that you are no longer baking their favorite holiday goodies, but if they participate in creating alternatives, they will be willing to support your recovery.

How to Say No to Your Family and Friends

Saying no to family and friends who encourage, nudge, or even push you to move away from your food plan is very hard. These friendly saboteurs often go right to the heart of your own ambivalence. You may have friends who insist you have a piece of birthday cake, or go to a Thai restaurant with them, or come over for a bite of the coffee cake they just baked.

How can you set your boundaries with these folks? How can you say no gracefully? There are two tasks for you in dealing with these folks. One is learning how to refuse gracefully; the other is understanding how your own ambivalence may affect the outcomes.

The Art of Graceful (or Humorous) Refusal

On the community forum, we came up with great list of ideas for coping with holiday meals. Laura's tips combine practical advice with humor and are especially helpful when you're trying to avoid alcohol and dessert! They truly offer wonderful options for saying no in a new way.

1. Matter-of-factly request a seltzer when the host asks what you would like. Throw a slice of lime in it. That way, it will look like what everyone else is drinking and they'll leave you alone.

2. If there's no seltzer, throw your lemon or lime slice in a glass of water with ice.

3. Throw your lemon or lime slice at anybody who inquires about your strange eating habits.

4. Deftly turn the conversation so you direct it back to the person who is inquiring about your "diet." "How come you don't eat sugar?" they ask. "I have found I feel better," you reply. "What about you? Are there any foods that you don't eat because you feel better without them?" (People love to talk about themselves!)

5. Disappear when dessert is served. Go to the bathroom for an especially long visit. Drop by the TV room and instantly get interested in whatever show the kids are watching. Suddenly develop the need to go out to your car and get that evening wrap because you are cold. Studiously start removing those tiny, natty little balls from your polyester evening gown.

6. When dessert is served, say, "Thanks, but the main course was so delightful I filled up on it. But I would love a cup of tea." (Hosts love to please their guests and will run to get whatever the guest asks for. So keep them busy and help them do their job as hosts.)

7. Be honest. Of course, you will become the center of attention and people will instantly feel guilty about the dessert they are about to put into their mouth and hate you for it! Expect glares and wicked looks behind your back. Shrug them off.

8. Tell your partner/friend/spouse that you need help at the party. Instruct him or her that when dessert comes, it is their job to stick to you like glue and divert the conversation away from you—even if they have to do the macarena without music or recite the Gettysburg Address.

9. Choose to eat dessert and feel miserable. Then let everybody know how you feel by having a blood sugar/beta-endorphin crash right in the middle of the living room. They'll never serve you dessert again. They'll never serve you again, period. But who needed them as friends anyway?

10. You could forewarn the hostess that you have some discomfort in this

area. Could you bring a dessert that is allowable to you but bring enough for everybody? Could the hostess say she made it so attention is off you? You can then smirk when the guests eat the dessert and gag because it is so, well, sugar-free.

11. Write to Miss Manners and send your letter by overnight mail. She will know how to advise a guest in this potentially volatile situation. Avoiding conflict at dinner parties is paramount to a successful, well-mannered evening, wouldn't you agree?

12. Don't go to the party.

13. At 8:00 P.M. announce that you have to get back to the facility; nightly check-in is mandatory by 8:30, as sugar addicts in your program need to be locked up for the night.

14. Go to the party virtually. Get the latest "See You See Me" computer program and appear on screen at appropriate moments. Tell them it's a new work project the boss asked you to do. Virtually eat dessert with them.

15. Wear a paper bag on your head. That is sure to get more attention than a little ol' diet thing.

16. Bring enough copies of this book so when somebody asks you to elaborate, you can put a book in her hand and walk away. Tell her the discussion group on brain chemistry will begin after dinner.

17. Wear a sign that says, "I do Kathleen's plan; wanna do it with me?"

18. As everyone else eats dessert, smoothly pull a baked potato out of your evening bag and ask someone to pass the salt and pepper, please.

19. Start boring them with personal stories of the difference between a beta-endorphin crash, a serotonin drop, and low-blood-sugar shakes. ("You know, last Wednesday when I had that beta-endorphin crash, I thought I was going to take my boss's head off, I was so irritable, but in retrospect it was probably low serotonin because I didn't have the impulse control necessary to stop, so I kept yelling . . . Though it could have been low blood sugar because I missed breakfast and had a mediocre lunch and got all light-headed and jittery.") When their eyes glaze over, you have created a safe space for yourself at the party. They will avoid you, of course, but the attention is off you.

20. Pre-print cocktail napkins with the sugar/carbohydrate content of everything being served that night (you'll need to coordinate with the hostess on this one). Then trip lightly from guest to guest, informing them what they're doing to their pancreas, using the napkin as a visual aid.

21. Invite Oprah. No one will even notice you're there.

You can add to or adapt this list to fit your own style and your own needs. Many in our community copied Laura's list and carried it with them to millennium parties.

Tips from the Field: You Can Go Home Again

My parents seem to feel personally rejected when I don't eat their food. My dad and I had a silly argument during a recent visit about real potatoes vs. fake potatoes. When I do succeed with my parents, it's because of two things: First, I bring my own food supplies to their house and park them right in the kitchen for all to see. Early in the day, I may ask my mom what she is planning for dinner. I ooh and aaahh over things, saying something like, "Mmmm, sounds great! How about if I steam some broccoli to go along with that?" She is always glad for the help, and what mother could resist their kid eating vegetables? It's when I let myself get emotionally wrapped up in their need to parent me that I get into trouble.

—M.

How Your Ambivalence Can Affect Your No

But let's take a look at how your own feelings toward sugar recovery can affect saying no. The "helpful" person urging you to have her coffee cake might be ignoring your "No, thank you" because she can sense you aren't fully committed to your program. A critical key to successfully saying no is getting your own feelings squared away. Once you are absolutely convinced that your recovery is more important to you than sweets, your friends and family will get the message clearly. This may take many months or even more. One of the markers for your own progress is the respect you command from those around you about the food. The more serious about it you become, the more they will honor your commitment.

Staying Out of Trouble

It's not only family and friends that can get us in trouble. Sometimes we do it to ourselves. That's why the best way to stay *out* of trouble is to know what people and places will get you *into* trouble. Let's look at slippery places first. They will be different depending on where you found your old comfort foods. Trouble spots can be bakeries, ice cream parlors, or coffee shops, but they can also be Italian restaurants or Jewish delis with lavish dessert cases. In fact, any place that has an old emotional cue (when you go there you always have their pie, or you used to go there with your dad and get ice cream) can be a trouble spot for you.

When you are just starting to stay off sugars, be vigilant and don't go into those shops or restaurants at all. Three or four months down the road, when your brain and body quiet down, you'll be able to go in those places without fear of immediately falling off the program.

Why? Your brain chemistry will change and those places won't trigger you anymore. Your brain will respond to the visual and smell cues differently. When something (like sweet food) is emotionally charged, you see it everywhere. By the same token, when things are not charged, you don't see them. For example, if you are primed (and thus craving sugar) and you go into Starbucks, all you will see are the cookies and pastries in the glass case. But if you are solid with your program, you will simply order a decaf latte and won't even *see* the stuff in the case.

Do you know what your trouble spots are? Ask yourself this:

"What are the places that I drift to under stress?" Make a note of them below.

Where do I go? (Be specific)	When and why do I go there?	What do I eat?

Getting Support

Getting a lot of support is key to your success with this program. Whether you have one sympathetic friend or family member, a buddy to do the program with, a large local support group, or the huge resources of online support on our community forum, you will find that support makes all the difference in sticking to your plan over time.

Getting Friends and Family to Help

Your new way of eating may have gotten you support from friends and family in the beginning, but you need support for the long term. This is best provided either by others who are on the program or by people who are not sugar addicts themselves. Here's an example. I went out to lunch recently with someone who is doing the program. Her partner came with us. We were at a restaurant that had really good bread. When the waiter came with a big basket of warm breads (you can be sure no browns were included) and a pair of tongs for serving it, the woman on the program said thanks, but she didn't want any. Her partner—who is *not* a sugar addict—also turned down the bread, not because she didn't want any, but as a gesture of support. I was very touched.

You can create your own little support group of people who are interested in what you are doing and who aren't in denial about their own sugar sensitivity. Ask your friends to exchange "safe" recipes. See if someone would like to do the program with you. Invite your group to one of the elegant dinners listed in Chapter 7. Have a potato taste-testing using white, yellow, Peruvian purple, Yukon Gold, and all the other varieties of potatoes now available.

Email one another, make phone calls, connect every day. This is important and will make a huge difference.

Online Support

You can find lots more support if you have access to the Internet. If you don't own a computer, you can try hooking in via your television set through Web TV, use a friend's computer, or see if your local library has Internet access for its patrons.

You can reach my Web site at www.radiantrecovery.com. There you will find an overview of the program along with answers to frequently asked questions, helpful hints, products to support your program, and other great resources like our newsletter, the community forum, a listing of local support groups across the country, and our special-interest online support groups. There is no charge for any of these services.

Tips from the Field: Using Online Support

This support is priceless. For me, it's the glue that holds the whole thing together.

—*L.*

Critical throughout this whole process is a commitment to getting support. You cannot heal addiction in isolation. Community moves you from self-sabotage into progress. It keeps you honest, encourages you, and delights in your success. Build your community and find what you want.

What to Do When You're Cranky

Even though you have a good support system, there will be times when you are cranky. "Cranky" is the code word that I use to describe the feeling of "wanting to kill!" The first step in dealing with cranky is to notice it when it comes up. The clues are that you will be edgy and irritable, feeling like everything and everyone are in your face.

When you notice this, go back to your food journal. Have you eaten something sweet, something that primed your beta-endorphin system and brought up cravings that are setting off your crankiness? Have you been eating enough? You may not be eating enough food at your meals or you may be skipping meals. Or your meals may be light on the protein. Also look to see if you are getting enough complex carbohydrates. Sometimes people just do protein and vegetables, and they get really cranky. Protein and veggies aren't enough. You have to eat some browns every day: whole grain bread, brown rice, beans, or any whole grain products. (If you are a One-Pot/One-Meal type, this means that every pot you cook will need to include browns.) And don't forget your evening spud.

The Way out of Cranky

The solution to cranky is very simple. Get back to the basics. Eat breakfast with protein. Eat three meals a day with protein. And be sure you are getting enough brown things. What's enough? Well, it's different things for different people.

If you are just getting off sugar, your meals will consist of protein, browns, and vegetables. The ratio of browns to greens will probably be two browns to one green. As you continue with the plan, the ratio will shift to about one to one. If you decide to use the plan to lose weight, you would shift to one brown to two greens. These shifts seem to occur spontaneously. When I wrote *Potatoes Not Prozac*, I didn't discuss this, but I have noticed that this is what people on the program usually do spontaneously.

You May Be More Sensitive to Sugar Now

When you first go off sugar, your brain and your receptors are going to be much more edgy and volatile. So if you have a little bit of sugar, you are going to feel it a whole lot more than you will after you've been on the program awhile and everything quiets down.

Here's the time frame we are talking about. For the first four months off sugar, you may feel euphoric and really excited about doing the program. You have gotten through your detox, which was uncomfortable but manageable, and overall you feel quite steady. From about four to seven or eight months, your brain chemistry quiets down and your receptors aren't so reactive, but they are now like newborns. They are very receptive and vulnerable to sugar. During this period of time, people may also have more food allergies. Their systems seem to be more reactive and volatile, even though they have changed their food dramatically. After eight or nine months, the entire system seems to quiet down and fall into a regular routine, and you'll be less vulnerable to slipping. If you slip a little, you won't slide down the entire mountainside. On a practical level, what that means is that if you do go to a party, it won't matter what they are serving. If you have to eat white things or even sweet things, it will be okay. You won't be severely triggered and you won't fall apart.

Tips from the Field: The Blessings of Time

Now that I have been on the program for fifteen months, I am much less sensitive to sugar than I was at three to nine months. It is like my body is now more grounded and absorbs the shock better. This doesn't tempt me to go back on my substances, but it does make for a smoother ride. My chemistry is not so volatile. It is more stable, so shocks don't shatter me; they just rock me a little and I can get back on track more easily.

—*D.*

Tips from the Field: The Bottom Line

If you remember nothing else, remember this: *Eating sugar makes you want more sugar.* Period. Early on in the process, I couldn't understand when people told me that "a little bit is harder than none." But it's true.

—*L.*

What About Relapse?

We talked in Chapter 6 about slipping and full relapse. Slipping is when you slip off the plan for a meal or two. Relapse is when your slip stretches into days or weeks or months. Relapse rarely descends on you from out of the blue. It is usually preceded by a number of slips and some clearly recognizable symptoms. The warning signs of relapse are:

Emotional fragility	Inability to concentrate
Fatigue	Irritability
Feeling on edge	Low tolerance for stress
Feeling inadequate	Thinking that goes round
General edginess	and round

Don't Expect Perfection

There is no such thing as perfection. Every one of us makes mistakes from time to time—and sometimes we make them frequently. We are not striving for perfection. We are seeking commitment and progress. Work to know what and why you are eating what you do. You may well choose a date to commit to going off sugars and into detox, but there is no magic date for being fixed in recovery from sugar addiction. The Sugar Addict's Total Recovery Program is not a short course in change. Rather than simply giving up sugars, you are working on a life plan.

If you set yourself to believe that you will be totally abstinent for the rest of your life, you are setting yourself up for failure. Doing this program doesn't work that way. It is a *process* of becoming more aware, more attentive, and more committed as you go. It is cumulative. That means it builds on itself over time. And it builds on the problem solving you do as you go.

As you learn to handle new situations, as you learn to recover from a slip, you will be smarter and savvier each time. Food will no longer be your enemy, but your support. Your body will be a trustworthy guide and you will be having fun with your life.

Tips from the Field: Making Better Choices

When I am tempted to eat sugar, I always picture a balance scale. On one side is how I feel now and how I hope to change, and on the other side is the piece of dessert or whatever choice I am facing at the moment. Then I ask myself: Is it worth giving up my contentment and emotional stability for this particular choice? For me, looking at it in that stark way really makes it clear exactly what I'm contemplating.

—L.

If You Fall Off Your Food Plan

When you feel your worst and can't cope with anything, just go back to eating breakfast every day with protein. As you start feeling better, expand to three meals a day with protein. And so on. Don't spend a lot of time or energy beating yourself up. Just pick up the program and get going again.

How to Get Back to Your Plan

How do you get back on the plan when you haven't just slipped, but have seriously relapsed? The answer is: Take a special day and pay attention. Eat three meals with protein at regular intervals, and record your food and feelings in your journal.

One client I see gets a fresh start by treating herself to three meals out. She has a fancy omelet with fresh fruit and whole wheat toast for breakfast, a Greek salad or Caesar salad with grilled chicken for lunch (she brings her own salad dressing to avoid covert sugars), and fish or beef as the main course for dinner. She says it's worth the expense to get herself back on her food plan without feeling deprived!

If you have been off the program for some time, you have some choices about how to get back on it. Some people like to start back in slowly, working their way up through the steps. Others jump back into a sugar detox. It's your own call.

Take Chris, for example. She had been doing the program for eighteen months when she really got into trouble. She ended up being off the program for three months. She was not able to control her eating and she was losing her grip. She was scared she might go back to being the way she was before she started dealing with her sugar addiction.

I recommended that she give herself three weeks to get fully back on the program. The first step was for her to reconnect to the Web community. Chris agreed. She knew she couldn't do it by herself. So she started posting and answering messages on the Community Forum. The next action I asked her to take was to move the chocolate she ate to mealtime.

After she had gotten this in place, I encouraged her to use bananas rather than chocolate, even if she had to eat three bananas a day. In this way, we created a banana "bridge" that would ease the pain of her detox. This is not something I would recommend to someone doing their first detox, but I recommended it with Chris because we wanted her to stop being primed by the emotional cues from the chocolate. She could cope with the sweetness of the banana. The bananas were sort of medicinal. (There's no way you can think of chocolate as medicinal!) They probably had almost the same amount of sugar in them, too, since Chris wasn't eating huge amounts of chocolate.

After a week, she found she didn't need the banana and got fully back on track. So she didn't end up needing the whole three weeks, but by permitting her to take that long if she needed to, I took away the emotional pressure.

Creating Other Kinds of Comfort

When you were regularly eating sweet food and foods made with refined flour in order to comfort yourself, you probably thought the only thing that could comfort you was sugar. But that was just your sugar-addicted body speaking. Now that you have shifted from white things, which are often high in sugar, to brown things, you may notice your mind opening to the possibility of other forms of comfort. This is a sign that sugar is losing its grip on you.

The comfort that sugar and white flour give you when you are feeling down is really our old friend the beta-endorphin spike, which makes you feel great for a moment, then sends you into beta-endorphin withdrawal—and creates huge cravings for more sugar.

Things That Will Trigger a Beta-Endorphin Spike

The danger of a beta-endorphin spike is that it *increases* your risk of slipping or relapsing. If you don't eat, if you skip a meal, you will get a beta-endorphin spike, which will prime your system and set you up for big cravings. If you have a wildly enthusiastic exercise session, the same thing can happen. One woman on the program told me that the day she started her Christmas shopping, she bought a lot of gifts, and that made her feel so good, she couldn't stop buying. Another example of beta-endorphin release.

Other things that can trigger a too-big beta-endorphin release are:

- Going into a casino and hearing coins jingle in metal cups
- Making love a lot all at once
- Going on a vision quest (coming down after a big high can make people have cravings)
- Staying up all night and cramming for an exam
- Having a baby

Do you get the idea? Going to extremes in a short period of time is going to flood your system with too much beta-endorphin. So watch out for activities of high intensity and short duration.

How to Get a Nice Slow Rise in Your Beta-Endorphin

When you use comfort foods and activities that produce a *slow* rise in beta-endorphin, you will feel better and keep feeling better. No rush, no withdrawal symptoms, no cravings.

The list of activities that have been scientifically documented to raise your beta-endorphin slowly includes meditation, yoga, exercise, prayer, music, eating food that tastes good (other than sweet or white-flour-based foods), making love, laughing, listening to Mozart and other classical music, and listening to inspirational talks. It's my guess that the complete list includes much more, even though these other things have not been tested in the laboratory or reported in the science literature. They include dancing, gardening, puppy kisses, kitty snuggles, children and grandchildren sleeping or running or laughing, bubble baths, candles, even going to the movies with a dear friend.

Our community has named these activities BE raisers, meaning beta-endorphin raisers. Make your own list. You may be surprised at the number of BE raisers you can find.

Tips from the Field: Lifting Your Spirits

Here are some of the things I do when I'm feeling really depressed:

- **Go to the park with a book (even if just for ten minutes)—it's good because it gets me out of the house.**
- **Go to the library and stay there long enough to read three magazines.**
- **Cook a pot of soup (all that chopping is very therapeutic!).**
- **Do a jigsaw puzzle.**
- **Go look in a pet shop (providing it's not near a doughnut shop!).**

—C.

Here are some beta-endorphin raisers that work for me:

- **Go watch a ball game in the local park—whichever teams are playing, kids or adults. (You don't have to know any of the players or even know what time the game started.)**
- **Clean off one surface in the house—maybe a table, a section of cabinet. Getting it to look its best, perking it up, brightens the whole room and me.**
- **If it's winter, build a fire, put on soft music, and curl up.**
- **Eat out on my balcony or have my morning quiet time there.**
- **Meet a friend out for coffee or a meal, with the motivation of having them really enjoy it (like they have been under stress lately).**
- **Go to a public event—any event—and participate as a spectator.**

—D.

Here are a few things I do to nurture myself in non-food ways:

- **Write poetry.**
- **Listen to *The Cowboy Junkies* or other favorite CDs.**
- **Meditate.**
- **Do deep-breathing exercises.**
- **Lift weights and stretch.**

—S.

Seems like whenever I need comfort or am stressed, I start heading for sweets or food! But I do have a few non-food things I've done that work for me.

- **Take a leisurely hot bath.**
- **Float in a pool, all by myself.**
- **Hug my bird.**
- **Call a dear friend from whom I haven't heard for a while.**
- **Put lavender essential oil on my pillow and down comforter, and take an afternoon nap.**

—L.

Here are some things that work for me. Maybe they will work for you.

- **Go back to reading *Potatoes Not Prozac*. Start at the beginning.**
- **Take a walk.**
- **Exercise.**
- **Watch a comedy-romance movie with a good friend you can snuggle up with.**
- **Go window shopping.**
- **Read a romance (or any other book of your choice).**
- **Go dancing!**
- **Review your journal just to see how far you've come along since the beginning and remember how it felt to be powerless over food.**
- **Go roller-skating just for the fun of it!**
- **Play board games with your friends and/or family.**
- **Go online and chat with someone on the community forum.**
- **Send an email to a close friend whom you haven't sent mail to in a while.**

Finally, remember to smile when you look at yourself in the mirror! You are your own best friend. *No one* can take better care of you than you. You know what is good and not so good for you. Choose what's best for you because *you deserve it*!

—*L.*

As you start to identify your personal beta-endorphin raisers, you are going to start connecting to the idea that life can be more than food. Growing up, many of us learned to get our comfort, safety, and security from what we ate. As adults, we don't realize that it isn't the food so much as the feeling associated with the food that makes us feel so good. The feeling is about beta-endorphin. Feeling safe, confident, and loved. Feeling connected. This is beta-endorphin.

Learning that we can have these feelings from a thousand things other than food is a wonderful insight. The quality of the beta-endorphin rise from puppy kisses is not as dramatic as that from an ice cream sundae, but it sure has a bigger upside to it. And the best part of beta-endorphin-raising activities is you can do a lot of them at once. Get in the tub, light a candle, make a cup of tea, get your cat on the windowsill, put on some wonderful music, and get your spouse or partner to rub your back. For a beta-endorphin boost, these things may well equal that of a hot fudge sundae—and you won't be hungover the next day.

10

Special Situations

Have you noticed that life rarely goes according to plan? This isn't necessarily a bad thing—many of the surprises we run into can be wonderful ones—but it can throw our program off if we aren't expecting them. In this chapter, I'll give you some help in planning for the unexpected and in adapting the program to your special needs if you are diabetic, pregnant, or a vegetarian, or you take antidepressants.

Making Contingency Plans

Most sugar addicts who have not started to heal do not plan much. We tend to be impulsive and call it spontaneity. This actually means we rarely think ahead. One of the real markers for your recovery is to begin to think about your food needs *before* you get into trouble.

That's why you must always have a contingency plan—no matter what your cooking style. If you are going to a potluck dinner, for example, make sure the dish you are bringing is something you can eat. That way, if every other dish is loaded with sugar or white things, you will at least get some dinner. (You'll also need to make sure everyone else doesn't finish off your dish before you get some!)

Other contingency plans are to keep your own protein snacks in the car or make sure you have a little bag of almonds in your purse so if you get stranded somewhere, you have something to tide you over. (For other suggestions, go back and take a look at the sections in Chapter 6 on foods to carry with you, what to do if you are over the cliff, and what to do if you miss lunch.) The key is to *think ahead* about the situations in which you might have difficulty getting the food you need and *plan* for them! Let's take a look at some of these special situations that call for a little planning.

Going Out to Eat

When you are eating out, you can eat in almost any restaurant, but you will need to follow a few ground rules in order to enjoy yourself and care for your sugar-sensitive body at the same time.

First, if possible, know the menu of the restaurant before you go in. Make sure there are foods you can eat. Ask the waiter not to bring the bread basket to your table. And don't peek at the dessert list when you are looking over the menu.

Focus on finding the most enjoyable food you can have. Ask the waiter to have the chef adapt an entrée to suit your needs. For example, you could ask for a baked potato instead of pasta. You could ask for a sandwich with whole wheat bread—or without bread! I have had cooks come up with the most delightful options in response to my requests.

Tips from the Field: Restaurants to the Rescue

When I am in danger of going off the plan, I drop everything and get myself to a restaurant. I am an expert now on which restaurants around here meet my needs. I don't hesitate to take something from home to combine with what I know they have. Sometimes I take my tuna and dump it on their beautiful salad. Sometimes I slip a piece or two of whole grain bread in a plastic bag so I can have bread with their meal or make my own sandwich with their fillings.

—D.

I love eating out on this plan. My favorite things to order for lunch are a chicken Caesar salad, a Cobb salad, or a chef salad. For days when I'm in a rush, I take a couple of whole wheat tortillas down to the Mexican food stand and ask them to make chicken burritos without rice on them. If I run out of whole wheat tortillas, I just order the same burrito, open it up, and eat the insides.

—M.

Dining Out for Business or Pleasure

When you go out for a meal, first of all, enjoy yourself—especially if you are someone's guest! Scan the menu and decide what your main dish—your protein—will be. Steer clear of pasta dishes (unless you ask for the pasta sauce to be put on a baked potato instead of pasta) and dishes without substantial protein. Then decide about the accompaniments. Most restaurants will offer salads and side orders of veggies you can eat. If not, ask them to *cook* you a side order of steamed or sautéed veggies. Many will be glad to do so.

Asking for What You Want at a Restaurant

Even if something you want is not on the menu, you can ask them to make it for you. I do this all the time. I look at the menu to see what ingredients are there. For example, they may be serving chicken with cherry wine sauce. Now, I know that this sauce won't work for me, but I also know that they have chicken in the kitchen. Or there may be a great pesto sauce being served on the meat-and-pasta dish. So I bravely say, "Would you be willing to ask the chef [or cook] if I might have some chicken with that pesto sauce?" I have never had anyone refuse me. If the chef is huffy about your choice, you can always simply ask to have the chicken broiled.

Other ideas? You can order a double serving of vegetables. You can ask for any sandwich on the menu and end the request with "without the bread" and a smile. Or you can ask them to put any of their protein things on any of their salads—such as adding shrimp to a Caesar salad. Simply tell them you will be happy to pay for it, smile, and assume they will accommodate your request.

Really Good Places to Eat Out

Eating out can be just as much fun on the program as it was before; you just need to know where to go. My favorites are fish or seafood restaurants, steakhouses, and grills.

Folks on our community forum have even found a lot of possibilities in fast food restaurants. Here are some things they recommend:

- Hamburgers or cheeseburgers with lettuce, tomato, and onion, but without the roll. (Throw it out. If you just leave it in the bag on your table, you'll probably pick at it.)
- Salad bars or side salads (be careful about the covert sugars in their dressings; try taking your own homemade salad dressing—it'll be tastier, too).
- Chicken or beef tacos on corn tortillas at Taco Time or Taco Bell; steak tacos at Taco Bell. Other Mexican fast foods that will work are pinto beans with cheese, fajitas on

a corn tortilla, and a taco salad (dump it out of its white flour shell and throw it out or it will call to you all through dinner).

- Roast chicken without the skin at Kentucky Fried Chicken. (They also have good steamed corn on the cob.)
- Baked potato with chili, cheese, and/or salad bar stuff on top of it (Wendy's and some other places). You can also tear up pieces of a hamburger and put that on top if there's no other protein available.
- Grilled chicken salads (at Wendy's and McDonald's). Order two if you're concerned about not getting enough protein.
- Chicken strip salad with an extra broiled chicken breast ("bird in a bag," they call it) and waffle fries, which have their skins on (Chik Filet).
- Chicken nuggets, though they are admittedly boring without the dipping sauce, plus they are breaded with white flour. But if you are desperate for protein, most fast food places have them.
- Fried chicken and green beans (Hardee's).
- Salads and sandwiches at Subway (in some areas they offer whole wheat rolls).

Foreign Food

Some foreign food is great for folks on the program. And some is not. Here's how to tell the difference.

Asian

Chinese restaurants tend to put sugar in everything. It's my experience that they may do so even if you ask them not to. If you taste Chinese food that's truly cooked without sugar, you will know immediately. It tastes completely different. My advice is to either stop going into Chinese restaurants or really learn which dishes are least likely to have sugar in them. If you have a special place that you want to keep on your list, develop a relationship with the staff. If you are a known quantity to the staff, they are more likely to honor your request for no sugar.

Thai food is also loaded with sugar. It's rare to find a Thai place that can serve you a dish without sugar, though you can always ask for steamed vegetables without sauce. Some folks have had luck with that.

Japanese food also has sugar in it, though way less than Chinese or Thai food. Even the sticky rice used to make sushi has sweetener in it. Now, I still eat sushi on occasion because I love it. Sushi once in a while works for me. I know that the morning after I have it, I may crave all sorts of things. And I just laugh at myself and remember that it is the sushi being seductive and I don't have to do anything in response to the cravings. But remember, I have been doing the program for eleven years. If you are just starting off, you may want to be more rigorous and not flirt with triggering yourself.

Indian

In general, Indian food is not a problem for folks on the program. In particular, Indian restaurants are wonderful with vegetables. What's more, curry evokes a positive beta-endorphin response because it is hot. You can feel relaxed and mellow and not be triggered.

Italian

Sometimes people on the program avoid Italian restaurants because of the pasta and bread, but the truth is, Italian restaurants can be great places to eat because they also have grilled fish and vegetables, wonderful salads, and antipasto. The key is to know what your choices are before you go in and to ask them not to bring the bread to the table. Try reading the menu before you are falling off the cliff. And take care about the bread. That warm, crusty bread calls to me big-time. I want to be sloshing it in the olive oil and garlic. But I ask them not to bring it. Its call is too intense.

Mexican

Mexican is a good alternative, though it is not long on vegetables outside chopped tomatoes and beans. Be sure to ask for corn tortillas (blue is even better) instead of white-flour tortillas, and skip the rice. Eat the beans—they are a tasty, slow brown. Also, chili is comforting—it's warm in your tummy, and if it's spicy hot, it too evokes another positive beta-endorphin response. The beta-endorphin response to the chili is why some of us go into withdrawal when we leave New Mexico for too long.

Further Plans for Special Occasions

Special occasions call for special skills in dealing with them. Whether you are faced with trying to stay on your plan during holidays, birthdays, plane trips, or long car rides, remember: You can do it! Here are some tactics you can use.

Holidays

Head your holiday crisis off before it happens. Here's the bottom line:

Emergency Preparation = A Successful Celebration

Holidays and other family celebrations are times of high stress, and your body may get thrown for a loop as much by the stress (even good things can be stressful!) as by an excess of sugar and white things. This means that the best defense is a good offense: Plan ahead and be careful to eat right and to journal every mouthful and every feeling as you approach periods of high stress (if you know about it ahead). This will help your body be well prepared to handle the foods and moods of the holidays.

Another tactic is to find out ahead of time what will be served so that you know what foods you will and won't eat when you get there. If there's not enough to fit your plan, ask if you can bring your favorite salad or side dish. If that won't work for your hostess, at least she will be forewarned about your passing up her dishes that contain sugar and white stuff.

Two other helpful hints are to eat something before you go so you are not famished if dinner is late, and to plan an after-dinner walk with people. That will raise your beta-endorphin level so you are feeling happy and solid when you sit back down at the table and watch other people eating sugary desserts. You could also bring a dessert that you know you can eat (see the recipes in Chapter 11).

Another idea is to go to a restaurant for your holiday meal where you can get exactly what you want and you aren't offending your hostess by not eating her pasta dish or homemade eight-layer lemon cake.

Or you could also skip the big meal altogether and create an alternative celebration. Christmas and Hanukkah, for example, could be about doing service (helping cook dinner at a soup kitchen for homeless people) instead of eating a fancy meal together. Many families have found renewed gratitude and joy in celebrating the holidays this way.

Go back to the opening of Chapter 9 and take a look at the brainstorming list that Gretel did about Christmas. How might you apply that tactic to other holidays and special events? Remember *food* is not love, *love* is love. We often use food to express our love, but there are other ways to express love as well. Here's a good example.

Every Valentine's Day, the chocolate ads shout, "Show her you love her!" and accompany their command by a photo of a huge heart-shaped box of chocolates. But think of all the other ways someone could express his or her devotion and celebrate a true holiday of the heart:

- Spend extra time with the one you love.
- Write her a love letter.
- Read love poems out loud to him.
- Go for a walk together and hold hands.
- Give his dog a bath.
- Wash, wax, and vacuum her car.
- Buy her flowers or lingerie.
- Cook her a meal that fits the plan.
- Bring him breakfast in bed every Sunday for a month.
- Make a collage of all the images that remind you of him.
- Prepare her a scented bubble bath with candles and background music, and then keep her company while she takes it. Scrub her back if she wants and wrap her in a thick soft towel afterward.

There are lots of ways someone can show his or her love for you without sending your blood sugar sky-high.

Birthdays

For me, five minutes in the mouth isn't worth it anymore. With that in mind, here's a story about food, birthdays, and love.

My birthday was coming. A dear and supportive friend offered to make a special birthday cake that would fit my food plan, using whole grains, a little molasses, and very little sweetness. Chewy, moist, and spicy was what we were aiming for. The recipe we were adapting came from Martha Stewart.

My friend, who doesn't actually cook very much, came to my house for the big cake-making day. She unpacked the ingredients she had purchased and lined them up on the counter with great ceremony. Then confusion set in. Every few minutes she appeared in the study, where I was working. "Why do I have to simmer the ginger?" "Do I really need to sift the oat flour?" "Is baking soda the same as baking powder?"

Eventually she had concocted a gooey brown mass and was ready to pour it into the cake pan. This generated another visit to the study. "Kathleen, it says to put it in six miniature bundt pans. What are bundt pans?" By this time I was laughing so hard, I could hardly stand, let alone find a bundt pan of any sort. But my neighbor, the baker, came to the rescue and found something she thought would do. We cooked the cake and sprung it from the pan.

Frankly, it looked a little strange, like something that had died or been in the refrigerator too long. My son said it resembled a mosquito disk. I wondered how we would manage to eat it.

Everyone else at my birthday party slathered ice cream over their portion of the mosquito disk. I used applesauce. The cake was pretty strange; actually it was awful, but the whole experience was so funny, I didn't really care that I didn't have real cake.

Tips from the Field: Friends Are Better Than Cake

It was a tradition at work to have a cake for the birthday person, as many jobs do. One birthday, everyone knew I was trying really hard to lose weight, so that year they made me a delicious fruit salad, with lots and lots of cut-up fresh fruit. They had "extras" to put with it, like whole grain crackers, yogurt, and cheeses. I truly did not miss the cake at all—nor did anyone else! There was not a crumb left after the party, unlike the times when we had to try to pawn off a half a cake on someone at the end of the day. I have always remembered this, because I actually *preferred* it to a birthday cake (and believe me, it takes a lot to make me choose fruit over cake), it was so delicious and refreshing. Most of all, it showed how much my friends cared about me and took my food plan seriously. Friends like that are priceless.

—L.

It's been many years since I have had a rich chocolate cake with white frosting on my birthday, but like I said, five minutes in the mouth isn't worth it anymore.

Don't let anyone tell you, "You won't miss it after a while." Of course you will. It's like losing a dear friend. But over time, things shift. Your attachment will move from the sugar (the cake) to the love (the people). The joy will be in the party, the celebration, family, and friends. The taste of cake won't be your standard of love. There was more love in that "mosquito disk" than any cake I have ever had.

Tips from the Field:
To Eat or Not to Eat . . . Birthday Cake

Whichever choice you make, it's a learning experience. Hurray if you choose not to eat the cake, but don't beat yourself up if you do choose to eat it. If you choose to eat it, think about all the times you ate cake without having the choice. Just the idea that you could ponder, take the time to make a decision—why, that's pretty amazing in itself. Remember all the times the cake plate was empty before we even had a chance to taste it—let alone decide whether or not to eat it? Now, before you so much as see or smell that cake, you are already ahead of the game!

—*P.*

Traveling

Business travel, more than business meals, poses a problem for me. The only solution is to have a plan. When my first book was published, I went on an extensive book tour. I had asked my publicist to make sure that the local person escorting me to and from the airport, book signings, and media interviews knew that eating a healthy lunch was critical to me.

Unfortunately, my very first book signing took place at lunchtime. My escort brought me a can of tuna fish and a can opener. It wasn't quite what I had hoped for. But I learned my lesson quickly. *Do not trust that anyone other than you will understand that meals on the road are very important.*

When I saw the tuna can, I should have sent my escort across the street to get me a cup of lentil soup, some whole grain toast, and a piece of fruit. I didn't, and by 3:00 P.M., when we were driving to my next appointment, I was falling off the cliff. I might have slipped if I had gone into a coffee shop at that point and seen all those goodies looking me in the eye. Don't let yourself get into a blood sugar crisis.

Identify the windows of time during which it is critical that you eat. Ask about the restaurants in the place you'll be. Always get protein at your meals. And make sure you get enough to eat. If you are hungry and you get tired, you'll lose it on your trip. Stay in hotels with room service, because they will always make you a baked potato. The server who brings it won't think you are strange, only that you know what you want.

If you get into trouble, find a fast food place. Know ahead of time which ones offer foods that will work for you. (Refer to the specific suggestions earlier in this chapter.) Maybe even keep a

---

Tips from the Field: Traveling Light

If you're traveling, it helps to take a small ice chest. I found one that is soft-sided and collapses when I'm not using it, so I can actually put it in a suitcase if it's empty. I got it at my local drugstore, of all places. It's easy to replenish the ice from hotel ice machines. If you are flying, you can pack it away and go to a grocery store to fill it up with food and ice when you get to your destination.

—K.

list of fast foods that fit your plan in your wallet so you don't have to wrack your memory when you're hungry and stressed.

And don't forget to write in your journal. Without it, I guarantee you won't be able to think straight or know what you have eaten when. Finally, cut yourself some slack. Traveling is stressful at best, and a lot of it is out of your control. Just do your best.

Surviving Long Plane Trips

Plane trips are a challenge! You can try ordering the special meals, but the best thing is to just bring your own food. Make a sandwich ahead of time and include cut-up veggies and some ranch dressing to use as a dip. Pack a salad, too, and bring some salad dressing in a little plastic bottle. Bring fruit, too, or whatever you think of as a treat. Maybe cheese and Triscuits. And bring *plenty* of food. Use plastic bags or old yogurt containers to pack your foods so you can toss them out when you reach your destination.

If you are on the return leg of a journey where you've been staying in a hotel, eat a solid meal before you leave and get the hotel restaurant to make you a whole grain sandwich—or whatever works for you—so you can take it on the plane with you.

Plan for the fact that you will get stuck in an airport that has minimal food options. I keep a packet of George's Shake with me whenever I travel. It has saved my blood sugar a number of times.

Eating in the Car

For the occasional meal in your car, you can use the suggestions in Chapter 6 on getting food in convenience stores and buying foods to carry with you. This advice also applies to car vacations, but in this case there are lots of other things you can do.

• Start your day with a George's Shake plus some breakfast food such as eggs, bacon, or sausage. You can pack the powder and a container in which to mix it, and order the milk and/or orange juice at the restaurant where you are stopping. Or carry the milk with you. If you are staying in a motel without a cooler, you can keep a pint of milk on ice overnight in an ice bucket in your room. It will melt, but the milk will still be okay in the morning.

• Don't rely solely on restaurants. Travel with a stash of emergency foods such as Triscuits, peanut butter, almonds, apples, and cheese. You can also get packages of four individual servings of unsweetened applesauce (if your market doesn't have them, look at a whole foods grocery). This is especially good with peanut butter, and for a treat for kids.

• Many grocery stores have good deli sections now, and often you can get half a chicken and some cooked vegetables for a decent price (and save tipping).

• Keep your eyes open for roadside fruit and vegetable stands. These aren't so easy to find since we are all driving the interstates now, but if you see one, you might stop for a stretch and pick up a fresh treat or two. Make sure to eat protein with your fruit—nuts or cheese or plain yogurt—if it is a snack.

• Don't forget Mr. Spud. You can get baked potatoes many places (including Wendy's). Order a take-out baked potato or wrap up part of the potato that came with your dinner in a napkin to eat later as your evening spud. You can sometimes get fries, home fries, potato salad, and even mashed potatoes with skins on. Just look around and be flexible.

• Make sure you plan ahead and bring whatever kitchen stuff you need: sharp knife, plastic bags, paper towels, baby wipes (for cleanup), silverware (or plastic), plastic cups, salt and pepper. Think about it and make up a little box of supplies.

• Remember when you are traveling that getting even a little dehydrated can lead to cravings. If you don't drink your water (or if you miss your evening potato or skimp on protein), I can almost guarantee you will go for the sodas or sweets when you pull in for a pit stop.

Also, stretching, fresh air, a change of position, a change of activities, and beta-endorphin raisers (ranging from a quick walk to watching the clouds drift by as you sit in a field dotted with wildflowers) will all help your chemistry stay up and stable.

Other Special Situations

Many people ask me what to do if they have a "special circumstance."

You Take Antidepressants

If you are taking antidepressants, this program is an ideal addition to your medication. Many people find that "doing the food" enhances the effectiveness of their meds. Talk with your doctor. Give him or her this book. Plan to spend at least six months being steady with your food before you even consider going off your medications. If and when you are ready to do so, talk with your doctor to plan a slow and reflective taper that fits your lifestyle.

You're a Vegetarian

A very active group of vegetarians is doing this program. It is absolutely possible to have a successful plan and retain your commitment to your vegetarian program. Here are suggestions from some of our folks.

Try some of the high-protein prepared foods you will find in the natural food stores. These include things like:

- Baked tofu, which comes in vacuum-sealed packages and quite a few different flavors (examples are Thai, smoked, teriyaki, barbecue)
- Tofu spreads or pates
- Seitan, which is wheat gluten and extremely high in protein

- Other imitation-meat items that you can find in the refrigerator case or in the freezer case, like sausages, bacon, bologna, and tofu hot dogs

Use tofu and tempeh and beans as your protein source. Tofu is really flexible. You can mash it and make burgers. You can cube it and sauté it with garlic and soy sauce. You can scramble it with an egg for breakfast. You can food-process it and add it to pancake or muffin batters. Check your local bookstore for cookbooks geared to tofu.

Tempeh is the more textured by-product of tofu making. It has chunks of soybean in it and a firm texture. Tempeh can be sliced into strips and sautéed with soy sauce and garlic, or you can marinate it in anything (for example, barbecue sauce) and bake it. These bars of flavored baked tempeh are firm enough to be used in sandwiches.

Get a good bean cookbook and learn to make different dishes. Bean spreads will probably be very useful to you—you can eat them on bread or crackers, or scooped up with pieces of green or red pepper (a favorite for me). The easiest bean spread/dip in the world is to take a can of drained black beans and put it in the food processor with a couple of tablespoons of your favorite salsa and maybe some extra red pepper flakes and garlic. If it isn't creamy enough, add a teaspoon or so of olive oil and blend again.

I think variety can be an issue, and if you do some of these plant-food alternatives, eggs and cheese will look less boring to you. The most important part will be to get creative and stay committed to maintaining the level of protein that will work for you.

You're Pregnant

If you are sugar sensitive and pregnant, this plan can truly enhance how both you and the baby feel during your pregnancy. There are a few simple precautions to remember. Do *not* do a fast detox. You may be impulsive and want to clear out all that sugar quick so you can get on with the program. But your baby should not do a quick detox under any circumstances! Do *not* go cold turkey. Ease into it. Substitute fruits for your typical sweet foods. Shift slowly.

You may also need to eat more frequently than the three meals a day I recommend. Plan to have a mid-morning and mid-afternoon snack with both protein and complex carbs. If you are getting nauseated, it often means that your blood sugar level has dropped. Your growing baby comes first and your body will give it your glucose first, leaving you going over the cliff. Do not let yourself get into an over-the-cliff state. Eat enough and eat frequently enough so that your blood sugar stays steady for both you and your baby.

You Have Diabetes

While this program was not originally designed for people with diabetes, it seems to have a very positive effect. Most of the diabetics we are working with have Type 2 diabetes, which means not only are their glucose levels high but the insulin doesn't work properly for them. Because simple carbs are converted very quickly to glucose, they can cause your glucose levels to rise very high. The brown and green (and yellow and red) carbs you will eat on the program will be far less likely to spike your sugar levels than the simple white carbs you may be most drawn to.

The combination of the protein at every meal and the slow carbs can make a huge difference for you. If you are working at controlling sugar levels with diet only, you need to be even more on top of what you eat than someone who is taking medication does. This program will give you guidelines and support for creating a plan that fits your needs. Not only will you tailor your plan to your style, but you can also factor in your own individual diabetes concerns. This is not a one-size-fits-all plan. It is your plan for your body.

Many diabetics are reporting their blood sugar levels going down and stabilizing as they do the program. If you are diabetic, however, it is better *not* to use a regular potato for your evening carb snack. Choose complex carbs that have a lower glycemic index such as sweet potatoes, whole wheat bread, or whole wheat crackers such as Triscuits. Visit my website for more information geared specifically to your needs.

Tips from the Field: From Someone Who's Been There

So you've been diagnosed with diabetes and you're a little bummed. I was too, but now I look at it as a blessing in disguise. My life did change, but for the better. I see richer, deeper colors now. Being a diabetic on this program is not different than being anyone else on it, except I pay attention to my sugar levels as well. That's the beauty of the program.

I eat three meals a day. Each meal contains protein and a complex carbohydrate. I eat a snack at night. I choose what is best for my blood levels.

I feel good now. I *feel* now. I'm not numbing myself with too much sugar and too much food. My blood sugar isn't so high that I'm constantly sleeping. It's in the normal range the majority of the time.

Just because you've been diagnosed with diabetes doesn't mean it's the end of your life. With this program, it's just the beginning of life.

—S.

In Closing

As we tie things up, remember that the most special situation to consider always is your sugar-sensitive body. All this work will have enormous gains for you. As you "do the food," you are going to reconnect with your birthright. You will remember creativity, humor, clarity, intuition, and power that you have long since disconnected from. For a while, you may struggle with the concept that "doing the food"—something so simple and so not sexy—could be so powerful. But you will keep coming back to it. And the more you do, the stronger you will get and the more powerful your recovery will be.

Before we move on to the recipes, I want to share with you a very inspiring letter I received. It sums up what we are seeking:

After eight months of living/breathing/eating the program, I am happy to report a very radiant recovery. Last week a friend I hadn't seen in a year ended her long rave about how great I looked with "I wouldn't have recognized you if I'd seen you on the street." While it's wonderful to know that I look so much better, what is truly remarkable is how I feel and how I function now.

- *Gone are the aches and pains. In their place, I feel a fluid motion and an increasing strength as I've come to actually look forward to exercising.*
- *Gone are the brain fogs and indecision. In their place is a renewed vitality, a sense that I can accomplish what needs to be done.*
- *Gone are the restless, sleepless nights. In their place is deep, comforting sleep—and only six hours instead of eight or nine.*

Freedom. Great word. I'm free from the addiction that took away my pleasure in life, that life, which caused me to obsess and hate myself. I'm free from an addiction that skewed my view of the world and my place in it.

So I look at sugar and I put it in my left hand. And I put life as I know it now in my right hand and I ask my higher self to choose. Freedom, radiance versus a Hostess cupcake and a lifelong addiction to sugar?

I did the sugar when I saw no other alternative, no other way to comfort myself. I did the sugar because I didn't know what else to do. Now I have a choice. And I've made that choice. I am on the other side and I like it here! At long last, life is good.

May your own recovery from sugar sensitivity bring you this same freedom and joy!

11

Recipes from
Fellow Travelers

These recipes have come from members of our community
forum, people like you who are sugar sensitive and who are
looking for simple solutions. The comments on the recipes
have come from your neighbors and friends.

You don't have to be a "Cooking" type to enjoy these recipes.
Some are so simple that even the most cooking-phobic of you
will be willing to give them a try. Many have been designed to
provide the simple nutrition-filled meals loved by "Functional/
Factual" and "I Don't Want to Change" types. "One-Pot" and
"Salad" types will also find treasures in here.

After you try them out, let us know what you think at www.
radiantrecovery.com.

Breakfast

Oatmeal Apple Pancakes

I love these pancakes. They make a great Sunday-morning breakfast—tasty, filling, and wholesome.

1½ cups oatmeal (not instant)
2 cups milk or buttermilk
3 eggs
2 tablespoons safflower oil
1 cup whole wheat flour
1 teaspoon baking powder
1 teaspoon cinnamon
1 cup chopped apples

Soak the oatmeal in the milk or buttermilk for 5 minutes. In a separate bowl, beat the eggs and oil. In another bowl mix the flour, baking powder, and cinnamon. Add the dry ingredients to the egg mixture, then stir in the oatmeal mixture and the apple. Lightly grease a griddle or frying pan and heat until a few drops of cold water sprinkled on the pan dance. Drop pancake batter ¼ cup at a time on the griddle. Bake and turn to bake on the other side. If you want a topping, try applesauce or one of the toppings suggested for cottage cheese–cinnamon pancakes, below.

Cottage Cheese–Cinnamon Pancakes

A great topping for these pancakes is to cook some frozen blueberries in a saucepan with a little water until they get syrupy. Or use one banana and some strawberries frothed and mixed together thoroughly with a simple hand mixer. Some folks also put sour cream or plain yogurt on top.

1 cup rolled oats
1 cup low-fat cottage cheese
2 egg whites
2 teaspoons vanilla extract
½ teaspoon cinnamon
  milk
  fresh or frozen fruit

Chop the oats in a blender or food processor; add the cottage cheese and blend until the mixture is smooth. Beat egg whites until fluffy. Add to oatmeal cheese mixture. Add vanilla and cinnamon. If the batter seems thick, thin it by adding a little milk. After blending, stir in pieces of fresh or frozen fruit. Bake on a nonstick skillet or lightly greased griddle over medium heat, dropping batter onto the griddle using 2 tablespoons batter per pancake. Turn when edges are lightly browned.

Yogurt Ricotta Delight

This is a quick, simple, and creamy breakfast for one. It is a mainstay for many of us.

½ cup nonfat plain yogurt
½ cup nonfat ricotta
½ cup fruit (strawberries, raspberries, blueberries, bananas, fresh or
  frozen but unsweetened)
7–8 unsalted almonds (raw or roasted)

Mix together yogurt and ricotta until creamy. Blend in fruit and enjoy! Add almonds for extra protein. Try a little vanilla, cinnamon, or nutmeg according to your preference.

Microwave Nut Butter Oatmeal

This one sticks with you all morning. This has been tested in our community and has been called "a must for the sugar-sensitive breakfast hater." It is equally yummy made with almond butter, cashew butter, or tahini (sesame butter). If you like this breakfast for one, you can keep Ziploc bags of premeasured oatmeal and peanut butter in the fridge so you can just grab one in the morning.

¼ cup uncooked rolled oats
½ cup milk
1 tablespoon nut butter, sugar-free and preferably organic*

Combine ingredients and microwave on high for 1 minute, 20 seconds. This comes out fairly thick and a little sticky, so if that's not your style, add some banana slices, apple chunks, or raspberries before microwaving to smooth out the consistency.

*I recommend using organic peanut butter because there is some concern about the degree of pesticide concentrations in ordinary peanut butter. You can find organic peanut butter at natural foods stores.

Easy Egg and Oat One-Pan Breakfast

Here is a breakfast recipe (for one) that is quick and tastes great! Some folks like it with plain yogurt on top. This is another one of those we all play with to add, subtract, and change to suit our taste.

2 eggs
¾ cup milk or yogurt
1 cup oats
1 small apple, diced
Nutmeg and cinnamon to taste

Preheat oven to 350° F. Beat the eggs well. Stir in milk. Add oats, apple, nutmeg, and cinnamon. Pour into a buttered (or sprayed) pie plate and bake 30 to 40 minutes, or until set.

Let stand 5 to 10 minutes.

Oatmeal Muffins

Thanks go to Allison for this recipe.

1½ cups whole wheat flour
 4 teaspoons baking powder
 ½ teaspoon salt
 ½ cup milk or soy milk
 1 egg, well beaten
 1 banana or 1 jar banana baby food
 1 heaping tablespoon organic peanut butter
 1 cup cooked oatmeal

Preheat oven to 400° F. Grease a 12-muffin pan.

Combine flour, baking powder, and salt. In a separate bowl, stir milk, egg, banana, and peanut butter into the oatmeal. Now stir the dry ingredients into the oatmeal mixture. Spoon into muffin cups and bake 20 minutes, or until brown.

George's Shake

Here's the basic recipe for George's Shake and a couple of variations that folks from the community have sent in.

2 cups milk, soy milk, or oat milk
 ½ cup fruit juice
 2 tablespoons protein powder (choose a sugar-free one)
 2 tablespoons oatmeal (not instant)

Put all the ingredients in the blender and blend on high for about a minute. If you do it for less time, you will be crunching oats at the bottom of your shake. If you prefer not to use milk in your shake, use water and a little juice. What makes this shake work as a great breakfast choice is that it combines nutritious foods with plenty of protein.

These two variations use the premixed version of George's Shake (orderable via the Web site at www.radiantrecovery.com or by calling 888-579-3970).

The frozen berries in this version make the shake really cold and thick.

¼ cup George's Shake mix
8 ounces milk
½ banana
   Some frozen unsweetened berries

Combine all ingredients in a blender until smooth.

Here's a nondairy version. It has lots of protein, fiber, phytochemicals, essential fats, and flavor. This texture will be much thicker. Add more soy milk to taste.

¼ cup George's Shake
1 cup soy milk
½ cup frozen unsweetened blueberries
½ cup water (or a little less if you like your shake thicker)
4 macadamia nuts

Combine all ingredients in a blender until smooth.

Lunch

Crustless Quiche

A slice of this quiche makes a great lunch—or breakfast. Have it with a salad and a slice of whole grain toast. You can add meat to it if you need more protein.

4 ounces grated cheese (use your favorite)
½ cup chopped onion
½ cup broccoli

6 eggs

⅓ cup milk

Preheat oven to 350° F.

Spray a glass pie plate with a little olive oil spray. Add cheese and veggies to pie plate. Beat eggs and milk until frothy and pour it over the cheese and veggies. Bake 35 to 40 minutes.

After the quiche has cooked and cooled, cut into 6 slices.

Potato-Crusted Quiche, With or Without Meat

The first version of this quiche calls for meat. A vegetarian version follows. This dish is delicious cold and reheats well in the microwave. The recipe comes from Shani.

CRUST

1 to 1¼ pounds potatoes (Yukon Gold are nice, or russet) sliced into
   ¼-inch-thick rounds

FILLING

   1 tablespoon olive oil

1½ cups chopped onion

1½ cups chopped green or red peppers (or a mixture of both)

   1 teaspoon Jamaican blend spices (or any spice you like)

   1 cup turkey sausage (maybe ½ to ¾ of a pound), pork sausage, or ham

   4 ounces (about 1 cup) grated cheese (mozzarella, cheddar, or a blend
     of mozzarella and Parmesan)

EGG MIXTURE

8 to 10 eggs (depending on how much room your fillings take up and how
     big your baking dish is). If you make the meat-free version below,
     use more eggs.

   ½ teaspoon ground black pepper

Preheat oven to 350° F. Spray 9 × 13-inch glass baking dish (a ceramic or metal dish will lengthen the cooking time, and may be more apt to stick) with vegetable oil spray.

Steam potato rounds until just tender, 6 to 10 minutes. Transfer to rack and cool (or rinse with cold water if pressed for time). Line prepared baking dish with enough potato rounds to cover, overlapping slightly.

Warm olive oil in frying pan over medium heat. Add onion, peppers, and spices and sauté 5 minutes or so. Add sausage and sauté until meat is just cooked through. Remove from heat and drain off any excess oil. Mix in cheese. Spoon mixture evenly over potatoes.

Whisk eggs and pepper in large bowl or blender. Pour egg mixture over filling mixture in dish. Top with a little more cheese, if desired. Bake quiche until set in center, about 35 to 40 minutes. Cool 20 minutes, then slice. Serve warm or at room temperature.

Here's the vegetarian version. Feel free to try any combination of veggies you like. Use the same crust and egg mixture and follow the same procedures for assembly as above.

FILLING
- 1 tablespoon olive oil (or spray)
- 1 cup chopped onion
- 1 cup chopped zucchini
- 1 cup chopped mushrooms
- 1 teaspoon thyme
- 4 ounces crumbled feta cheese (plain or the tomato-basil feta)

Tofu Scramble

This nicely spicy dish comes from Zoe. You can mix the spices up in bulk beforehand and keep them handy for a super-quick meal.

- 1–2 tablespoons vegetable oil
- 8 ounces tofu
- ¼ cup water

Cooked vegetables, like sliced onions, peppers, zucchini, broccoli, and/or yellow squash (optional)

SPICE MIXTURE

1 teaspoon turmeric

1 teaspoon cumin

1 teaspoon curry powder

4 teaspoons onion powder

4 tablespoons nutritional yeast

4 teaspoons dried chives

4 teaspoons dried parsley

1 teaspoon sea salt

Heat oil in a large skillet. Mash and cook the tofu, stirring, for 2 to 3 minutes. Add ¼ cup water and 2 to 4 tablespoons of the spice mixture.

Stir and cook for 2 to 3 minutes. Add cooked vegetables (optional) before serving.

Feta-Walnut Spread for Veggies or Sandwiches

This is a great spread to take to a party. If you like strong cheeses, it's to die for. This spread is good on crackers or pita, or stuffed into celery. Also very nice with sliced ripe tomatoes on the side, or ripe cherry tomatoes. The recipe comes from Aliza Grayer Earnshaw.

1 8-ounce package feta cheese

⅔ cup shelled walnuts

¾ to 1 cup plain nonfat yogurt

1–2 cloves garlic (to taste), peeled and put through a press

Fresh ground pepper (to taste)

2 pinches marjoram

Break up feta into a food processor. Process until finely crumbed and put into a bowl. Now process walnuts until finely crumbed, and add to the cheese. Be careful with the walnuts—if you process them too long, they will become a paste. If you like added texture, reserve a few nuts and chop to a rougher texture, then add to the finer walnut and cheese crumbs. Mix all the crumbs together with a wooden spoon until well blended.

In a separate bowl, combine ¾ cup of the yogurt, the crushed garlic, the coarsely ground black pepper, and the marjoram. Now add the feta-walnut mix. Add more yogurt if you want the mix to be more like a dip than like a spread. Once you reach the consistency you like, add just a little more yogurt—about a heaping tablespoon. The mixture will thicken in the refrigerator, as the chopped walnuts absorb liquid from the yogurt.

Feta Frittata

This is a great way to get a good serving of veggies and protein together. It is surprisingly quick, and tastes great cold tucked inside a buttered pita, for lunch. It also reheats nicely. This recipe comes from Aliza Grayer Earnshaw.

Note: You can substitute spinach for the greens, but you will then need more than 4 cups, as it shrinks more. It also requires less cooking time than chard or kale.

¼ to ⅓ **pound tofu**

      A few shakes of soy sauce (I prefer shoyu—it's milder)

4 **eggs**

2–4 **tablespoons water**

About 4 **cups of greens such as kale, chard, or mustard greens, or a combination**

      Olive oil

1 **large clove of garlic (or several small cloves)**

      Red pepper flakes or black pepper to taste

2 or 3 **ounces crumbled feta**

Preheat oven to 400° F.

Drain the tofu and mash with a fork in a bowl or on a plate. Shake some soy sauce on it, so the tofu is dark in places, but don't saturate the tofu with the soy sauce. If you use shoyu, you can use more of it; if using conventional soy sauce, use less—it's very salty.

In a separate bowl, beat the eggs with water. Chop the greens. Heat a 10-inch iron skillet and pour in enough olive oil to coat the bottom and sides of the pan. Swirl it around once the pan has heated up.

Chop garlic (or put through a garlic press) and add it to the oil. Then add the chopped greens, cover the pan, and reduce the heat to medium-low. After a few minutes, uncover the pan and stir the greens down, adding a dash or two of red or black pepper to taste.

Now add the tofu and stir everything together. Lower the heat, and spread the mixture evenly over the bottom of the skillet. Arrange the crumbled feta evenly over the top. Slowly pour in the beaten eggs, being careful not to disturb the crumbled feta.

Turn off the burner and put the skillet into the preheated oven. Bake until set, about 10 to 18 minutes. It's okay for the frittata to brown on top.

Turkey Burgers

Turkey patties are pale and, to some people, unappealing in taste and appearance. Fixing them using this recipe from Terri solves that problem, and they taste really good. Even people who don't like mustard have liked these. Try eating the burgers in a whole wheat pita with onions, topped by a cucumber/yogurt mixture (kinda like a gyro).

¼ to ⅓ cup low-sodium tamari sauce (found in your Asian food section)

2–3 tablespoons stone ground mustard

20 ounces ground turkey, formed into 5 patties (or 5 frozen ground turkey patties, thawed overnight in the refrigerator)

In a 10- to 12-inch skillet over medium-low heat, mix together tamari sauce and mustard. Place turkey patties into the sauce. Turn patties to coat both sides, then cook without a lid over medium heat until done.

Variations: You can press minced onions into the patties before putting them in the pan and/or melt shredded cheese on top just before they're done.

Asian Salad

This recipe, from Zoe, is a great way to get your veggies. Feel free to experiment with the ingredients!

SALAD

½ head bok choy, sliced thin

4 green onions, sliced

1 cup bean sprouts

½ package grated carrots (or 3 carrots, grated)

½ package broccoli slaw

DRESSING

¼ cup rice vinegar

¼ cup soy sauce

¼ cup orange juice

2 teaspoons sesame oil

Pinch cayenne

Salt if desired

Combine all vegetables in a bowl. Mix together the ingredients in the dressing, pour it over the vegetables, and toss.

T 'n' T Salad

This easy salad from Terri is attractive—and very satisfying on a warm day. Serves two.

> 1 can water-packed solid white tuna
> Approx. 1 cup cottage cheese
> ½ to 1 tablespoon mayonnaise
> Dill to taste (optional)
> 1 whole tomato per person
> Salt and pepper

Drain liquid from tuna. Place in bowl and flake apart with a fork. Mix in enough cottage cheese to at least double your volume (do this to your taste preference). Add mayo and a sprinkle of dill to taste. Mix thoroughly. Set aside.

Wash a whole tomato and then slice off the stem end. Set aside. Scoop out the tomato's seeds and pulp, leaving the shell intact. Mix the seeds and pulp into the tuna and cottage cheese; season with salt and pepper to taste.

Fill the tomato shells with the mixture, mounding it up above the top of the shell, then place the stem-end slice of the tomato back on top like a jaunty cap. Serve with Triscuits.

Simple Tofu Salad

This recipe allows you to experiment on your own with ingredients and amounts.

Tofu
Mayonnaise
Mustard
Chopped pickles
Salt and pepper to taste

Mash up tofu with mayo and mustard, add pickles, salt and pepper. That's it! You can also add chopped celery or what else appeals to you. Be creative!

Chili Layered Casserole

This recipe from Laurie W. is way easy and it makes a lot. It also tastes great the next day.

1 package of fresh corn tortillas (*not* tortilla chips)
3 to 4 cans of turkey or chicken chili without sugar
4 cups shredded cheese (your choice of cheese, or use a combination of cheddar and Monterey Jack)

Preheat oven to 350° F.

Tear up tortillas into small bite-sized triangles. Put a layer of these tortilla triangles across the bottom of a 9 × 14-inch pan. Spoon a layer of chicken or turkey chili over the tortillas. On top of the chili, sprinkle shredded cheese, as much or as little as you like.

Repeat the layers of tortilla, chili, and cheese once more—or even twice if your pan has room. Bake 30 minutes or until cheese gets bubbly. Let cool for 15 minutes before cutting and serving.

Beef Chili

Here's a rich and satisfying chili from Jeanie that her family raves about. She tops it with chopped onions and grated cheese and serves with homemade cornbread.

1 pound ground beef, browned
1 onion, chopped
1 to 3 cloves garlic (according to your taste), minced

Red, yellow, and/or green peppers (or green chilies), chopped (optional)

1 15-ounce can chopped tomatoes

1 15-ounce can tomato sauce

3 or more tablespoons of chili powder, to taste

2 teaspoons cumin

2 or 3 28-ounce cans of pinto beans—or whatever kind of beans you like

Brown ground beef in a skillet, then add onion, garlic, and peppers. Sauté until vegetables are soft. Add tomatoes, tomato sauce, chili powder, and cumin and simmer for 30 minutes to 1 hour. Add pinto beans and let simmer for 20 minutes or so to let flavors mix.

Dinner

Roast Sticky Chicken

This recipe from Marie is a great way to roast a large chicken. It is reminiscent of those rotisserie-style chickens that are so popular now, and it is surprisingly easy to make. The meat comes out very moist and flavorful, so leftovers taste as good freshly cooked. Once you try it, you will never roast chicken any other way. Note: You need to season the chicken overnight, and baking time is 5 hours.

1 large roasting chicken, as big as you can find

4 teaspoons salt

2 teaspoons paprika

1 teaspoon cayenne pepper

1 teaspoon onion powder

1 teaspoon thyme

1 teaspoon white pepper

½ teaspoon garlic powder

½ teaspoon black pepper

1 cup chopped onion

In a small bowl, thoroughly combine all the spices. Remove giblets from chicken, rinse out the cavity well, and pat dry with paper towels. Rub the entire spice mixture into the chicken, both inside and out, making sure it is evenly distributed and down deep into the skin. Put the chicken in a zippered bag, seal, and refrigerate overnight.

When ready to roast chicken, preheat oven to 250° F. Stuff the cavity with the chopped onion and set in a shallow baking pan. Roast uncovered for 5 hours (yes, 250° for 5 hours).

After the first hour, baste the chicken occasionally (every half hour or so) with pan juices. The pan juices will start to caramelize on the bottom of pan and the chicken will turn golden brown. If the chicken contains a pop-up thermometer, ignore it.

Let chicken rest about 10 minutes before carving.

Chicken Roasted with Garlic

Here's another great spice combo from Marie for roast chicken. Note: You can put a whole peeled onion and 3 to 5 peeled cloves of garlic in the cavity instead of using onion and garlic powder in the spice mix.

- 1 large roasting chicken
  Olive oil
- 1 teaspoon garlic powder
- 1 teaspoon onion powder
- 1 teaspoon salt
- ½ teaspoon ground pepper
- 1 teaspoon paprika
- 1 teaspoon either fresh or dry basil
  Dash of cayenne or chili powder

Remove giblets from chicken, rinse out the cavity well, and pat dry with paper towels. Rub the chicken down with some olive oil to prevent dryness.

Mix spices together in a bowl and rub this mixture on the chicken. At this point, you may let the chicken marinate in its spices for a few hours or go ahead and roast it.

Cook chicken at 300° F. for one hour, then lower oven to 200° and cook for another hour.

You can make some dressing with garlic and stuff the bird.

Kathleen's Roast Chicken with Vegetables

This is how I like to do my chicken. It makes the veggies especially delicious.

1 roasting chicken (4–5 pounds)
6 garlic cloves, peeled
8 carrots, peeled and quartered
4 potatoes, peeled and cut in quarters

Preheat oven to 425° F.

Rinse chicken and pull skin away from breast. Insert garlic between skin and breast. Re-cover with skin.

Fill roasting pan half full with water.

Place chicken upright on chicken roasting stand (you can get these at specialty hardware or cooking stores). Put carrots and potatoes in pan.

Cook for 45 minutes. Reduce heat to 300° F. and cook another 20 to 30 minutes, depending on size of bird. Add more water as needed to pan.

When done, remove chicken and veggies. Make gravy from the juice in the pan. (If you don't know how to do this, look in any basic cookbook.)

Beef Stew

This is a great basic beef stew recipe, which comes from Barbara. You can dress it up if you want by adding lots more garlic and pa-

prika, plus frozen corn and frozen peas. Note: If you cook this in a Crock-Pot, all you need to do is coat the beef with the flour, put it in the Crock-Pot, then add all the other ingredients on top of it. Cook for 4 to 5 hours on high or 8 to 10 hours on low.

If you don't have a Crock-Pot, see the instructions below.

2	pounds beef, cut in chunks or cubes for stew
1 to 2	tablespoons whole wheat flour
2	tablespoons olive oil
3	potatoes with skins, cubed
4	carrots, cut in quarters
2	onions, sliced
3	stalks celery, cut in chunks
1	teaspoon salt
1	teaspoon pepper
2 or more	cloves garlic
1	teaspoon paprika
1	can crushed tomatoes (optional)
	Liquid as needed (V8 juice, more crushed tomatoes, or tomato sauce)

Coat the meat in the flour and brown it in the olive oil. Then add the other ingredients above plus enough liquid to cover. Cook covered on low heat for 1 to 2 hours. Optional: To spice this up, add lots of garlic and some more paprika.

Kathleen's Meatloaf

This was my first meatloaf recipe thirty years ago, and I am still quite fond of it.

MEATLOAF

½	pound ground beef
½	pound ground pork
1	cup old-fashioned oatmeal (not instant)

   2 eggs
   2 tablespoons toasted onion flakes
   ½ cup spaghetti sauce (I use one that has no sugar)

TOPPING
   ½ cup spaghetti sauce
   ½ cup water

Preheat oven to 350° F.

Grease a loaf pan with olive oil. Combine meatloaf ingredients and put them in the pan. Pour the other ½ cup spaghetti sauce and the water on top.

Bake 45 minutes to an hour or so, depending on how you like meatloaf. (I like mine crispy, so I let it cook longer, until it gets a little dark on the edges.)

Jeanie's Meatloaf

Here is a very moist and juicy meatloaf recipe from Jeanie. She recommends serving it with a big pile of mashed potatoes with the skins on and lots of fresh veggies.

      ½ pound of leanest ground beef you can get
      ¼ cup whole wheat bread crumbs
      2 eggs
      4 ounces tomato sauce
      ½ green pepper, chopped
      ¼ pound chopped mushrooms
 1 or 2 medium carrots, chopped
      1 medium onion, chopped
 ¼ to ½ teaspoon thyme
 ¼ to ½ teaspoon marjoram
      ½ teaspoon basil
         Salt and pepper to taste

Preheat oven to 375° F.

Mix all ingredients together and put into a loaf pan. Bake at 375° F. for about an hour.

Chicken Meatloaf

If you've never tried ground chicken, here's your chance. (It's delightful in burgers, too.) This recipe is from Allison.

Taco seasoning to taste (use one of the brands that has no sweeteners, like Bearitos)
⅓ cup mayonnaise (use sugar-free mayo if you are concerned that regular mayo will trigger you)
20 ounces ground chicken
1 16-ounce can black beans, drained
1 onion, grated
½ cup salsa, or to taste

Preheat oven to 350° F.

Mix taco seasoning into mayonnaise. Combine all ingredients in a bowl. Put in a loaf pan and bake for 1 hour.

Soy Meatloaf

This vegetarian recipe is courtesy of Betty and her husband. It is also good cold or warmed the next day in sandwiches.

1 package soy meat crumbles, thawed (found in freezer section)
2–3 eggs
1 cup of whole grain crackers or rolled oats
Onions, chopped (we like lots of onions, but adjust amount to your taste)
Salt and pepper to taste

Preheat oven to 350° F.

Dump everything into a bowl and mix (using your hands works best). If the mixture feels a little dry, add a tablespoon of water or olive oil. Form into a loaf or just press into a loaf pan and cover with foil. Bake 30 to 45 minutes, or until the center is hot. (Remember, this isn't meat you are trying to cook; soy crumbles come cooked.)

Italian Frittata

This is delicious, and you can add extra protein (and moistness) to it by adding cottage cheese to the egg mixture. The recipe comes from Zoe.

2 tablespoons olive oil
1 cup sliced fresh mushrooms
1 cup zucchini, sliced
½ red bell pepper, sliced
½ green bell pepper, sliced
1 scallion, chopped
1 garlic clove, minced or pressed
6 eggs
3 tablespoons Parmesan cheese
   Freshly ground pepper to taste
   Dash dried basil
   Dash dried oregano
3 tablespoons water

Heat the olive oil in a large skillet. Add mushrooms, zucchini, peppers, scallion, and garlic. Cook, stirring occasionally, until vegetables are tender, about 5 minutes.

While vegetables are cooking, combine eggs in a bowl with 1 tablespoon of the Parmesan. Add remaining seasonings and water. Pour mixture over cooked vegetables in pan. Loosely cover and cook over medium heat until eggs are set, 6 to 8 minutes. Sprinkle with the remaining Parmesan and a dash of paprika.

Salmon Patties

This recipe is from Robin, who recommends freezing some for quick meals. She says they are great with a baked red potato and fresh or frozen green beans.

- 1 small can skinless, boneless salmon
- 1 egg
- ¼ cup minced red onion
- 1 teaspoon crushed parsley
- 1 teaspoon crushed rosemary
- 1 piece whole wheat or spelt bread, crumbled

Mix all ingredients together. Form into three good-size patties. (They won't hold together too well at first, but they will get firmer as they cook.) Fry them in a lightly oiled skillet.

Baked Chicken and Lentils

Allison, who created this recipe, says there is a wonderful broth at the bottom of the casserole when it is done. You can either eat the broth with the dish or use it for something else.

- 4 medium carrots, thinly sliced
- 1 cup chopped onion
- 1 14-ounce can chicken broth
- 2 bay leaves
- 1 teaspoon salt
- ½ teaspoon poultry seasoning
- ⅛ teaspoon pepper
- 1 cup dry lentils
- 2½–3 pounds of chicken parts (breasts, thigh, drumsticks, and/or wings)

Preheat oven to 350° F.

Mix everything but the chicken together in a 3-quart covered casserole and bake for 15 minutes, covered.

Brown the chicken in a lightly oiled skillet. Place on top of the lentil mixture and bake for 1 hour, or until lentils and chicken are done.

Corn and Bean Hash

This satisfying dish from Allison has some neat texture contrasts. The celery and corn are crispy, the beans are soft and creamy, and the TVP soy granules are sort of chewy.

1 cup beef (or vegetable) broth
1 cup TVP (textured vegetable protein) soy granules (available in health food stores)
1 onion, chopped
2 stalks celery, sliced
1 clove garlic, minced
1 tablespoon olive oil
1 16-ounce can black beans, drained
1 16-ounce can pinto beans, drained
1 16-ounce can corn or 1 package frozen corn
   Salsa to taste
   Chili powder to taste
   Spike to taste
   Any other seasonings you fancy

Bring broth to a boil and mix in soy granules. Cover and set aside.

Sauté onion, celery, and garlic in oil until onion starts to brown. Add beans and corn and stir. Then add seasonings to taste. You'll need to experiment, but that's part of the fun!

Now stir in the soy granules and broth. Heat, stirring constantly, until heated through and until flavors have mixed together.

Bread, Soup, and Side Dishes

Spelt and Flaxseed Bread

Cheryl says this bread is a wonderful beta-endorphin raiser! Spelt flour is good for people with wheat allergies or intolerance. It is a very old grain in the same family (Triticum) as wheat. It is also lovely to work with, and its flavor is exquisite. For more information on spelt, do a search on the Web.

  1 tablespoon quick-rising yeast
1¾ cups warm water
  1 tablespoon honey (to help activate yeast)
  2 tablespoons vegetable oil
  4 cups spelt flour plus ¼ to ½ cup, reserved
  2 teaspoons dry milk powder
  2 teaspoons salt (optional)
  ¼ cup whole flaxseed

Dissolve yeast in warm water. Add honey and oil and mix well. Allow to sit until foamy. Mix together 2 cups of spelt flour, milk powder, and salt. Now add yeast liquid to dry ingredients. Stir well (some folks use their hands). Add flaxseed. Mix well. Add remaining 2 cups of flour and mix until dough ball forms.

Use some of the reserved flour to dust a bread or cutting board and lightly knead until smooth and elastic. Shape and put in an oiled or Pam-sprayed loaf pan. Let rise until doubled.

Bake at 350° F. for 45 to 50 minutes, or until done.

Cool in pan on rack for 10 minutes. Remove loaf from pan and let cool completely.

Great Potato Soup

Here is a great soup recipe from Cheryl. She sometimes uses it as her nighttime "spud."

  2 tablespoons olive oil
  ¼ cup chopped onion
  2 cloves minced garlic
  ½ teaspoon whole cumin seeds
  1 tablespoon whole wheat flour
1¼ cups milk, divided
  1 large baking potato, cubed and boiled (do not peel)
  1 cup water
  1 tablespoon dilly mustard
    Salt and pepper to taste

Heat 1 tablespoon olive oil in nonstick frying pan.

Add onion and cook until soft.

Add garlic and cumin seeds, cook until slightly browned (not too long, as they will become bitter). Remove to saucepan.

Add second tablespoon of olive oil to frying pan and heat. Add 1 tablespoon flour to make roux.

After browning, add ¼ cup milk to make white sauce, and cook over medium heat for 10 minutes until thick and bubbly. Add onion mixture in saucepan along with potato, the rest of the milk, and water.

Bring to a gentle boil and add mustard. Stir to blend. Add salt and pepper and cook for 15 minutes.

Roast Potatoes

These potatoes are one of my favorites.

2½ pounds white or russet potatoes
1 teaspoon garlic powder
2 tablespoons toasted onion powder
1 teaspoon basil, fresh chopped
  A little salt and pepper
1 tablespoon olive oil

Preheat oven to 350° F.

Slice potatoes lengthwise in strips. Mix all remaining ingredients in a plastic bag. Shake the mixture and add the potatoes to coat.

Place on a baking sheet that has been covered with foil. Bake skin sides down for approximately 30 minutes.

Roasted Lemon Potatoes

Here is another potato option from Marie. These are great!

5 medium potatoes
  Juice from 1 large lemon
1½ tablespoons dried oregano
4 tablespoons olive oil
½ cup water
  Black pepper to taste

Preheat oven to 375° F.

Cut potatoes into small to medium chunks. Put in 13 × 9-inch baking pan sprayed with cooking spray.

Mix all other ingredients together and pour over potatoes. Mix together well.

Bake until done, approximately 1–1½ hours, stirring every 15 minutes.

Spicy Oven-Fried Potatoes

Marie keeps us from getting bored with our potatoes.

6–8 medium potatoes, cubed
  3 tablespoons olive oil
  ½ teaspoon salt
  ¼ cup Parmesan cheese
  2 teaspoons garlic powder
  1 teaspoon paprika
  ¼ teaspoon cayenne pepper
    Black pepper to taste

Put potatoes in large bowl. Pour olive oil on potatoes and stir to coat.

Mix all other ingredients together and pour over potatoes. Stir well.

Place potatoes in 13 × 9-inch pan sprayed with cooking spray. Roast in oven for 1–1½ hours or until tender and brown, stirring occasionally.

Stir-Fried Lemon Asparagus

This is a great dish for when company comes. It was sent in by Tammy.

2 pounds asparagus
2 tablespoons sesame oil
2 cloves garlic, minced
1 8-ounce can water chestnuts, drained
1 chicken or vegetarian bouillon cube (preferably without MSG)
3 tablespoons fresh lemon juice
2 teaspoons grated lemon rind
3 teaspoons soy sauce
  Salt and freshly ground black pepper to taste

Wash and dry asparagus and break off the tough part of the stems. Cut diagonally into 2-inch pieces.

Heat oil in a nonstick frying pan or wok over medium-high heat. Stir-fry garlic for 1 minute. Add asparagus and water chestnuts. Stir-fry for about 3 minutes. Add bouillon cube, lemon juice, lemon rind, and soy sauce.

Cook another minute or so until asparagus is crisp-tender and all ingredients are heated through.

Season with salt and pepper to taste. Serve immediately.

Larry's Famous Green Beans

This recipe comes from Aliza Grayer Earnshaw.

    2 pounds fresh green beans
    7 Roma or Italian tomatoes
  2–4 tablespoons extra-virgin olive oil
    1 large or several small cloves garlic
      Salt and black and red pepper
    1 teaspoon dried marjoram
    ½ teaspoon dried basil
    1 onion, thinly sliced into rounds (optional)
      Juice of 2 small lemons

Wash, top, and tail beans, and break into halves or thirds. Trim stem point from tomatoes, and chop the tomatoes in food processor or chop finely by hand.

Heat olive oil in deep skillet or casserole. Press or mince garlic, and sauté in oil until just brown. Add salt, pepper, and chopped tomatoes. Let simmer a few minutes, then add herbs and green beans. Add thinly sliced onions, if using. Stir everything together, cover, and simmer on medium to low heat, stirring a few times so beans don't stick to the bottom.

Cook until the beans are nicely soft, but not falling apart. They should still have shape and texture. When beans are tender, add the lemon juice, stir, and check for seasoning. You can add more salt, pepper, or lemon juice to taste.

Serve warm or cold.

Note: Instead of marjoram and basil, you can use fresh basil only (lots), or tarragon and basil.

Kathleen's Apple Carrots

This is one of my favorites.

   8 carrots
   Olive oil for sautéing
   ½ cup apple juice
   ½ cup water

Peel and slice carrots. Sauté in olive oil until browned. Add apple juice and water. Bring to a simmer and cook until soft.

Scalloped Cabbage

This is one of Cheryl's delicious recipes. Even if you are not a big fan of cabbage, I recommend trying it at least once.

   1 head of cabbage, sliced into thin strips
   1 10¼-ounce can cream of mushroom soup
   1 cup whole grain cracker crumbs (like Triscuits)*
   2 tablespoons butter
   3 tablespoons milk

Preheat oven to 350° F.

Boil cabbage until tender. Drain and put in 1½-quart casserole. Stir in remaining ingredients. Cover and bake for 35 to 45 minutes.

*Make cracker crumbs by breaking up crackers into small chunks and placing between two sheets of waxed paper. Roll with a rolling pin to crunch the bits down to crumb size.

Fried Eggplant with Yogurt-Garlic Dressing

This recipe comes from Susan S., who writes: "One of the joys of having a Turkish husband is learning 101 ways to cook eggplant—it is practically the national vegetable of Turkey. Eggplant is wonderful in texture and can make a very convincing substitute for meat. This is my favorite eggplant recipe—and my simplest."

1 medium eggplant
  Olive oil for sautéing, as little as possible

DRESSING
1 cup plain yogurt
  Minced or pressed garlic to taste
  Salt to taste

Preheat oven to 350° F. Slice the eggplant into 1-inch-thick slices, either width-wise or length-wise, whichever you prefer. Roast in the oven until slightly golden in color and slightly tender. Then fry in olive oil.

Whip yogurt until smooth and add garlic and salt. Top with dressing.

Oven-Fried Sweet Potatoes

This is a recipe for one, suggested by Cheryl. Try this as your before-bed potato. If you want to make these as part of a meal, figure one potato per person.

1 sweet potato
  Vegetable oil
  Salt and pepper to taste
  Onion powder to taste
  Garlic powder to taste

Wash and peel the potato, then cut it into french fry–size pieces. Put a little oil on a cookie sheet or in the tray of your toaster oven, and dump the fries on it. Turn them to coat all sides with oil. Then sprinkle with salt, pepper, onion powder, and a little garlic powder. (Or substitute nutmeg for onion and garlic powders.)

If you are using a conventional oven, bake at 450° F. for 15 minutes, turning once so the bottoms don't burn.

If you are using a toaster oven, bake at 425° F. for 20 minutes, turn them (the bottoms get nicely brown), then turn off the oven and let them sit for another 10 minutes.

Sweet Potato Puff

This recipe from Jeannie D. has gotten rave reviews everywhere, but remember, because of the eggs, you can't use this dish for your nightly spud. Also, you will need to experiment with the amount of nutmeg, as it tends to be quite overpowering if you use too much.

3 or 4 medium sweet potatoes
    1 teaspoon baking powder
       Dash of cinnamon or more, to taste
       Dash of nutmeg or more, to taste
    3 eggs
    1 tablespoon butter

Puncture sweet potatoes with a fork, then bake in a 350° F. oven for an hour, or until fork-tender. Take them out and immediately peel them. (You will find that when they are still hot, the skin virtually falls off.) Chop them up roughly and put them in a food processor with baking powder, cinnamon, nutmeg, eggs, and butter. Process right away (so the heat from the potatoes doesn't get a chance to cook the eggs) until the mixture is as smooth as baby food.

Place mixture in an ovenproof pan sprayed with Pam and bake at 350° F. for about 30 minutes. The puff will be soufflé-like. Watch it to make sure the edges do not get overly brown. When you spoon into it, it will collapse (like it's supposed to!).

Sweet Potato Pie

Cheryl makes a sweet potato pie by adding the sweet potato puff recipe to a whole wheat piecrust.

Fried Brown Rice with Onions, Almonds, and Cumin

This recipe from Cheryl makes enough for one serving. Multiply it if you are cooking for others. It's best eaten immediately, as the lovely crunchy browned almonds go soft after a short while.

- 1 tablespoon butter
- ¼ onion, chopped
  Small amount slivered almonds
- 1 cup *cooked* brown basmati rice
- ½–1 teaspoon ground cumin (to taste)

Melt butter in a nonstick fry pan. Add onion and nuts and cook until the onion is translucent and the nuts are browned. Add precooked (or leftover) rice and cumin, and cook until warmed through.

Salad Dressings

Basic Vinaigrette

Here's one to experiment with. It is good for marinating cooked veggies, and I put it on my potato.

- 4 tablespoons cold-pressed extra-virgin olive oil
- 2 tablespoons balsamic vinegar
- 1 teaspoon toasted garlic flakes
- 1 teaspoon grated fresh ginger
- 1 teaspoon dried orange peel

Combine all ingredients and shake. It tastes even better the next day.

Simple Salad Dressing

My favorite salad dressing.

- ⅓ cup fresh lemon juice (1 large or 1½ small lemons)
- ¾ cup olive oil (or sometimes I mix canola and olive)
- 1–2 tablespoons tamari soy sauce
- 2 large cloves garlic, crushed
  Fresh ground black pepper to taste

Shake all ingredients in a bottle.

Treats and Desserts

Squash Pie with Peanut Butter Glaze

Allison sent in this wonderful dessert recipe.

- 1 acorn squash
- ½ cup tofu
- ½ cup organic peanut butter
  Juice from ½ orange
  Cinnamon
  Nutmeg
  Ground ginger
  Whole wheat pie shell, purchased or homemade

TOPPING

- 1 tablespoon butter
- 1 tablespoon peanut butter
  Grated rind from the same ½ orange

Cut squash in half, remove seeds, and bake on greased cookie sheet at 350° F., skin up, until it's soft. Scoop flesh out of skins into bowl. Add tofu, peanut butter, and orange juice. Mix with electric beater until well blended. Add cinnamon, nutmeg, and ground ginger to taste. Fill pie shell with mixture and bake at 350° F. for 30 minutes.

When pie is nearly cool, heat topping ingredients in small saucepan, stirring constantly to prevent burning. Pour over pie. Refrigerate and serve cold.

Carrot Cake

This recipe comes from Allison.

1½ cups grated carrots
 2 eggs
 ½ cup oil
 1 jar banana baby food
 1 cup whole grain flour (wheat, oat, rice, etc.)
 1 teaspoon baking soda
 1 teaspoon cinnamon
 ½ teaspoon salt

FROSTING
 1 8-ounce package cream cheese
 ¼ teaspoon lemon extract
 1½ teaspoons vanilla extract

Preheat oven to 350° F.

Combine carrots, eggs, oil, and baby food in a large bowl. In a smaller bowl, mix together flour, baking soda, cinnamon, and salt. Then stir these dry ingredients into the carrot-egg mixture. Pour into greased 8-inch square pan. Bake 30 minutes, or until toothpick comes out clean.

While cake is cooling, combine frosting ingredients and adjust seasonings to taste. Frost when cake has cooled.

Pumpkin Tofu Cheesecake

Another creation from our dessert queen, Allison.

CRUST

1½ cups crumbs from whole grain crackers such as Triscuits or Wasa multigrain

⅓ cup melted butter

FILLING

12 ounces silken tofu

1 cup canned pumpkin

1 jar banana baby food

1 teaspoon cinnamon

½ teaspoon cloves

4 ounces cream cheese

1 tablespoon vanilla extract

Make crust first. Combine cracker crumbs and butter and press into pie plate. Pre-bake crust at 350° F. for 10 minutes, or until lightly browned. Set aside.

In a blender, combine filling ingredients, blend well, then pour into crust. Bake for 1 hour at 325° F., or until knife comes out fairly clean and middle is not liquid. Cool overnight before serving.

Pumpkin Cake with
Cashew Butter Frosting

Here's an interesting dessert variation that Allison came up with.

1¾ cups whole grain flour (try a mix of oat and brown rice flour)

 3 teaspoons baking powder

 ¾ teaspoon salt

 1 tablespoon cinnamon

 1 tablespoon nutmeg

 1 teaspoon allspice

 1 teaspoon ginger

 2 eggs, beaten

 ½ cup oil

 1 cup canned pumpkin

 ⅓ cup water

 1 jar banana baby food

FROSTING

 Cashew butter

Preheat oven to 350° F.

Stir together flour, baking powder, salt, and spices. In a separate bowl, mix eggs and oil. In another large bowl, combine pumpkin, water, and baby food. Add egg mixture to pumpkin mixture. Then add to dry ingredients and stir until well mixed. Pour into greased 8-inch-square pan and bake for 30 minutes, or until toothpick comes out clean.

Cool, then frost with cashew butter and enjoy.

Ricotta Fruit "Pudding"

This is a lovely dessert for one. Feel free to substitute other dried or fresh fruit for the dried apricots. Allison sent in this one.

3 dried apricots

3 almonds

¼ cup ricotta cheese

Couple of drops of vanilla, almond, or orange extract (optional)

⅛ teaspoon (or less) cinnamon or a dash of grated lemon rind (both are optional)

Chop the apricots and almonds into small pieces and mix into the ricotta cheese along with (optional) the vanilla extract (or whatever other flavor you may have chosen). Microwave on high for one minute. Top with cinnamon or lemon rind.

Bibliography

Abrahamson, E.M., and A.W. Pezet. *Body, Mind and Sugar.* New York: Holt, 1951.

Anderson, I.M., et al. "Dieting reduces plasma tryptophan and alters brain 5-HT function in women." *Psychol Med* 20(4): 785–791, 1990.

Arem, R. *The Thyroid Solution.* New York: Ballantine, 1999.

Barnard, R.J., et al. "Effects of a high-fat, sucrose diet on serum insulin and related atherosclerotic risk factors in rats." *Atherosclerosis* 100(2): 229–236, 1993.

Beattie, M. *Codependent No More.* Center City, MN: Hazelton, 1992.

Bertoli, A., et al. "Differences in insulin receptors between men and menstruating women and influence of sex hormones on insulin binding during the menstrual cycle." *J Clin Endocrinol Metab* 50(2) 246–250, 1980.

Besson, A., et al. "Effects of morphine, naloxone and their interaction in the learned-helplessness paradigm in rats." *Psychopharmacology* (Berlin) 123(1): 71–78, 1996.

Black, B.L., et al. "Differential effects of fat and sucrose on body composition in A/J and C57BL/6 mice." *Metabolism* 47(11): 1354–1359, 1998.

Blass, E.M. "Interactions between contact and chemosensory mechanisms in pain modulation in 10-day-old rats." *Behav Neurosci* 111(1): 147–54, 1997.

Blass, E., E. Fitzgerald, and P. Kehoe. "Interactions between sucrose, pain and isolation distress." *Pharmacol Biochem Behav* 26: 483–489, 1987.

Blass, E.M., and A. Shah. "Pain-reducing properties of sucrose in human newborns." *Chem Senses* 20(1): 29–35, 1995.

Blass, E.M., and D.J. Shide. "Opioid mediation of odor preferences induced by sugar and fat in 6-day-old rats." *Physiol Behav* 50: 961–966, 1991.

Bowen, D.J., and N.E. Grunberg. "Variations in food preference and consumption across the menstrual cycle." *Physiol Behav* 47: 287–291, 1990.

Brewerton, T.D., et al. "Comparison of eating disorder patients with and without compulsive exercising." *Int J Eat Disord* 17(4): 413–416, 1995.

Brown, G. "CSF serotonin metabolite (5-HIAA) studies in depression, impulsivity, and violence." *J Clin Psychiatry* 51(4; suppl.): 31–41, 1990.

Brown, R. *An Introduction to Neuroendocrinology.* Cambridge: Cambridge University Press, 1994.

Brunani, A., et al. "Influence of insulin on beta-endorphin plasma levels in obese and normal weight subjects." *Int J Obes Relat Metab Disord* 20(8): 710–714, 1996.

Bujatti, M., and P. Riederer. "Serotonin, noradrenaline, dopamine metabolites in trancendental meditation-technique." *J Neural Transm* 39: 257–267, 1976.

Christie, M.J., and G.B. Chesher. "Physical dependence on physiologically released endogenous opiates." *Life Sci* 30(14): 1173–1177, 1982.

Cleary, J., et al. "Naloxone effects on sucrose-motivated behavior." *Psychopharmacology* 176: 110–114, 1996.

Cronin, A., et al. "Opioid inhibition of rapid eye movement sleep by a specific mu receptor agonist." *Br J Anaesth* 74(2): 188–192, 1995.

Czirr, S.A., and L.D. Reid. "Demonstrating morphine's potentiating effects on sucrose intake." *Brain Res Bull* 17: 639–642, 1986.

Dalvit-McPhillips, S.P. "The effect of the human menstrual cycle on nutrient intake." *Physiol Behav* 31: 209–212, 1983.

de Waele, J.P., K. Kiianmaa, and C. Gianoulakis. "Distribution of the mu and delta opioid binding sites in the brain of the alcohol-preferring AA and alcohol-avoiding ANA lines of rats." *J Pharmacol Exp Ther* 275(1): 518–527, 1995.

de Waele, J.P., et al. "The alcohol-preferring C57BL/6 mice present an enhanced sensitivity of the hypothalamic beta-endorphin system to ethanol than the alcohol-avoiding DBA/2 mice." *J Pharmacol Exp Ther* 261(2): 788–794, 1992.

DesMaisons, K. *Biochemical Restoration as an Intervention for Multiple Offense Drunk Drivers.* Diss. The Union Institute. Ann Arbor: UMI, 1996. 9704758. www.libumi.com/dxweb/results

———. *Potatoes Not Prozac.* New York: Simon & Schuster, 1998.

Dienstfrey, H. *Where The Mind Meets the Body.* New York: HarperCollins, 1991.

Drewnowski, A. "Why do we like fat?" *J Am Diet Assoc* 97(7; Suppl.): S58–62, 1997.

Drewnowski, A., and C.L. Rock. "The influence of genetic taste markers on food acceptance." *Am J Clin Nutr* 62(3): 506–511, 1995.

Drewnowski, A., and R.C. Greenwood. "Cream and sugar: Human preferences for high-fat foods." *Physiol Behav* 30: 629–633, 1983.

Drewnowski, A., C.L. Kurth, and J.E. Rahaim. "Taste preferences in human obesity: Environmental and familial factors." *Am J Clin Nutr* 54(4): 635–641, 1991.

Drewnowski, A., et al. "Diet quality and dietary diversity in France: Implications for the French paradox." *J Am Diet Assoc* 96(7): 663–669, 1996.

———. "Naloxone, an opiate blocker, reduces the consumption of sweet high-fat foods in obese and lean female binge eaters." *Am J Clin Nutr* 61(6): 1206–1212, 1995.

Drewnowski, A., and J. Holden-Wiltse. "Taste responses and preferences for sweet high-fat foods: evidence for opioid involvement." *Physiol Behav* 51(2): 371–379, 1992.

———. "Changes in mood after carbohydrate consumption." *Am J Clin Nutr* 46: 703, 1987.

Dufty, W. *Sugar Blues.* New York: Warner, 1975.

Eades, M.R., and M.D. Eades. *Protein Power.* New York: Bantam, 1996.

Eipper, B.A., and R.E. Mains. "The role of ascorbate in the biosynthesis of neuroendocrine peptides." *Am J Clin Nutr* 54: 1153S–1156S, 1991.

Fantino, M., J. Hosotte, and M. Apfelbaum. "An opioid antagonist, naltrexone, reduces preference for sucrose in humans." *Am J Physiol* 251(R): 91–96, 1986.

Fernstrom, J.D., and D.V. Faller. "Neutral amino acids in the brain: Changes in response to food ingestion." *J Neurochem* 30: 1531–1538, 1978.

Fernstrom, J.D., and R.J. Wurtman. "Brain serotonin content: Physiological regulation by plasma neutral amino acids." *Science* 178 (Oct. 27): 414–416, 1972.

———. "Brain serotonin: Increase following ingestion of carbohydrate diet." *Science* 174 (Dec. 3): 1023–1025, 1971.

Fernstrom, J.D., F. Larin, and R. Wurtman. "Correlations between brain tryptophan and plasma neutral amino acid levels following food consumption in rats." *Life Sci* 13: 517–524, 1973.

Fernstrom, J.D., Ph.D. "Acute and chronic effects of protein and carbohydrate ingestion on brain tryptophan levels and serotonin synthesis." *Nutr Rev* 1986 May; 44suppl: 25–36.

———. "Dietary amino acids and brain function." *J Am Diet Assoc* 94: 71–77, 1994.

Fernstrom, M.H., and J.D. Fernstrom. "Large changes in serum free tryptophan levels do not alter brain tryptophan levels: studies in streptozotocin-diabetic rats." *Life Sci* 52(11): 907–916, 1993.

———. "Brain tryptophan concentrations and serotonin synthesis remain responsive to food consumption after the ingestion of sequential meals." *Am J Clin Nutr* 61: 312–319, 1995.

Forsander, O.A. "Is carbohydrate metabolism genetically related to alcohol drinking?" *Alcohol Alcohol* 1: 357–359, 1987.

Fredericks, C. *Carlton Fredericks' New Low Blood Sugar and You.* New York: Putnam, 1987.

Free, V., and P. Sanders. "The use of ascorbic acid and mineral supplements in the detoxification of narcotic addicts." *Journal of Orthomolecular Psychiatry* 7(4): 264–270, 1978.

Froehlich, J.C., et al. "Importance of delta opioid receptors in maintaining high alcohol drinking." *Psychopharmacology* 103: 467–472, 1991.

Frye, C.A., and G.L. Demolar. "Menstrual cycle and sex differences influence salt preference." *Physiol Behav* 55(1): 193–197, 1994.

Genazzani, A.R., et al. "Central deficiency of beta-endorphin in alcohol addicts." *J Clin Endocrinol Metab* 55(3): 583–586, 1982.

Gentry, R.T., and V.P. Dole. "Why does a sucrose choice reduce the consumption of alcohol in C57BL/6J mice?" *Life Sci* 40: 2191–2194, 1987.

Giannini, A., et al. "Symptoms of premenstrual syndrome as a beta-endorphin: two subtypes." *Program Neuropsychopharmacol Biol Psychiatry* 18(2): 321–327, 1994.

Gianoulakis, C., and J.P. de Waele. "Genetics of alcoholism: Role of the endogenous opioid system." *Metab Brain Dis* 9(2): 105–131, 1994.

Gianoulakis, C., et al. "Endorphins in individuals with high and low risk for the development of alcoholism," in *Opioids, Bulimia, and Alcohol Abuse and Alcoholism,* L.D. Reid, ed. New York: Springer-Verlag, 1990, 229–247.

Gianoulakis, C., B. Krishnan, and J. Thavundayil. "Enhanced sensitivity of pituitary beta-endorphin to ethanol in subjects at high risk of alcoholism." *Arch Gen Psychiatry* 52(3): 250–257, 1996.

Gianoulakis, C., et al. "Different pituitary beta-endorphin and adrenal cortisol response to ethanol in individuals with high and low risk for future development of alcoholism." *Life Sci* (England), 45(12): 1097–1109, 1989.

Goas, J.A. "Endocrine factors underlying the ethanol preference of rodents." *Pharmacol Biochem Behav* 10(4): 557–560, 1979.

Goldman, J.A., et al. "Behavioral effects of sucrose on preschool children." *J Abnorm Child Psychol* 14(4): 565–577, 1986.

Gosnell, B.A., et al. "Centrally administered mu- and delta-opioid agonists increase operant responding for saccharin." *Pharmacol Biochem Behav* 45(4): 979–982, 1993.

Gosnell, B.A., and D.D. Krahn. "The relationship between saccharin and alcohol intake in rats." *Alcohol* 9: 203–206, 1992.

Grau, J.W., R.L. Hyson, and S.F. Maier. "Long-term stress-induced analgesia and activation of the opiate system." *Science* 213(18): 1409–1410, 1981.

Greden, J. "Anxiety or caffeinism: A diagnostic dilemma." *Am J Psychiatry* 131(10): 1089–1092, 1974.

Hall, F.S., et al. "Effects of isolation-rearing on voluntary consumption of ethanol, sucrose and saccharin solutions in fawn hooded and Wistar rats." *Psychopharmacology* (Berlin) 139(3): 210–216, 1998.

———. "The effects of isolation-rearing on sucrose consumption in rats." *Physiol Behav* 62(2): 291–297, 1997

Harte, J.L., et al. "The effects of running and meditation on beta-endorphin, corticotropin-releasing hormone and cortisol in plasma, and on mood." *Biol Psychol* 40(3): 251–265, 1995.

Heitkamp, H.C., et al. "Beta-endorphin and adrenocorticotrophin after incremental exercise and marathon running—female responses." *Eur J Appl Physiol* 72(5–6): 417–424, 1996.

Heller, R., and R. Heller. *The Carbohydrate Addict's Diet.* New York: Dutton, 1991.

Hetherington, M., and J. MacDiarmid. "Chocolate addiction: a preliminary study of its description and its relationship to problem eating." *Appetite* 21: 233–246, 1993.

Holt, S., et al. "A satiety index of common foods." *Eur J Clin Nutr* 49: 675–690, 1995.

Hong, S.M., et al. "Self-esteem: the effects of life-satisfaction, sex, and age." *Psychol Rep* 72(1): 95–101, 1993.

Ipp, E., R. Dobbs, and R.H. Unger. "Morphine and beta-endorphin influence the secretion of the endocrine pancreas." *Nature* 276: 190–191, 1978.

Israel, K.D., et al. "Serum uric acid, inorganic phosphorus, and glutamic-oxalacetic transaminase and blood pressure in carbohydrate-sensitive adults consuming three different levels of sucrose." *Ann Nutr Metab* 27: 425–435, 1983.

Jenkins, D.J.A., et al. "Slowly digested carbohydrate food improves impaired carbohydrate tolerance in patients with cirrhosis." *Clinical Sciences* 66: 649–657, 1984.

Jias, L.M., and G. Ellison. "Chronic nicotine induces a specific appetite for sucrose in rats." *Pharmacol Biochem Behav* 35(2): 489–491, 1990.

Kampov-Polevoy, A.B., et al. "Association between preference for sweets and excessive alcohol intake: a review of animal and human studies." *Alcohol* 34(3): 386–395, 1999.

———. "Suppression of ethanol intake in alcohol-preferring rats by prior voluntary saccharin consumption." *Pharmacol Biochem Behav* 52(1): 1–6, 1994.

———. "Evidence of preference for a high-concentration sucrose solution in alcoholic men." *Am J Psychiatry* 154(2): 269–270, 1997.

Kanarek, R.B., and N. Orthen-Gambill. "Differential effects of sucrose, fructose and glucose on carbohydrate-induced obesity in rats." *J Nutr* 112: 1546–1554, 1982.

Kanarek, R.B. "Does sucrose or aspartame cause hyperactivity in children?" *Nutr Rev* 52(5): 173–175, 1994.

Keim, N.L., et al. "Effect of exercise and dietary restraint on energy intake of reduced-obese women." *Appetite* 26(1): 55–70, 1996.

Kinsbourne, M. "Sugar and the hyperactive child." *N Engl J Med* 330(5): 355–356, 1994.

Kirkby, R.J., and J. Adams. "Exercise dependence: the relationship between two measures." *Percept Mot Skills* 82(2): 366, 1996.

Krahn, D.D., et al. "Fat-preferring rats consume more alcohol than carbohydrate-preferring rats." *Alcohol* 8(4): 313–316, 1991.

Krauchi, K., et al. "High intake of sweets late in the day predicts a rapid and persistent response to light therapy in winter depression." *Psychiatry Res* 46(2): 107–117, 1993.

Kuzmin, A., et al. "Enhancement of morphine self-administration in drug naive, inbred strains of mice by acute emotional stress." *Eur Neuropsychopharmacol* 6: 63–68, 1996.

Laeng, B., K. Berridge, and C. Butter. "Pleasantness of sweet taste during hunger and satiety: effects of gender and sweet tooth." *Appetite* 21: 247–254, 1993.

Leibach, I., et al. "Morphine tolerance in genetically selected rats induced by chronically elevated saccharine intake." *Science* 221: 871–873, 1983.

Lloyd, H.M., et al. "Acute effects on mood and cognitive performance of breakfasts differing in fat and carbohydrate content." *Appetite* 27(2): 151–164, 1996.

Lowinson, J., P. Ruiz, and R. Millman, eds. *Substance Abuse: A Comprehensive Textbook,* 2nd ed. Baltimore: Williams & Wilkins, 1992.

Macdiarmid, J., and M. Hetherington. "Mood modulation by food: an exploration of affect and cravings in 'chocolate addicts.' " *Br J Clin Psychol* 34 (Pt1): 129–138, 1995.

Mann, P.E., G.W. Pasternak, and R.S. Bridges. "Mu 1 opioid receptor involvement in maternal behavior." *Physiol Behav* 47(1): 133–138, 1990.

Mathews-Larson, J., and R.A. Parker. "Alcoholism treatment with biochemical restoration as a major component." *International J of Biosocial Res* 9(1): 92–106, 1987.

McDonald, R.B. "Influence of dietary sucrose on biological aging." *Am J Clin Nutr* 62(1 Suppl.): 284S–292S; discussion 292S–293S, 1995.

McGuire, W.J., et al. "Enhancing self-esteem by directed-thinking tasks: cognitive and affective positivity asymmetries." *J Pers Soc Psychol* 70(6): 1117–1125, 1996.

Morley, J.E., and A.S. Levine. "Stress-induced eating is mediated through endogenous opiates." *Science* 209(12): 1259–1260, 1980.

———. "The role of the endogenous opiates as regulators of appetite." *Am J Clin Nutr* 35: 757–761, 1982.

Moyer, A.E., and J. Rodin. "Fructose and behavior: does fructose influence food intake and macronutrient selection?" *Am J Clin Nutr* 58(5): 810S–814S, 1993.

Muller, B.J., and R.J. Martin. "The effect of dietary fat on diet selection may involve central serotonin." *Am J Physiol* 263(3 Pt 2): R559–R563, 1992.

Palmer, L.K. "Effects of a walking program on attributional style, depression, and self-esteem in women." *Percept Mot Skills* 81 (3 Pt 1): 891–898, 1995.

Panksepp, J., R. Meeker, and N.J. Bean. "The neurochemical control of crying." *Pharmacol Biochem Behav* 12: 437–443, 1979.

Parekh, P.I., et al. "Reversal of diet-induced obesity and diabetes in C57BL/6J mice." *Metabolism* 47 (9): 1089–1096, 1998.

Paul, G.L., et al. "Preexercise meal composition alters plasma large neutral amino acid responses during exercise and recovery." *Am J Clin Nutr* 64 (5): 778–786, 1996.

Pennington, J.A. *Food Values of Portions Commonly Used.* Philadelphia: J. B. Lippincott, 1994.

Pierce, E.F., et al. "Beta-endorphin response to endurance exercise: relationship to exercise dependence." *Percept Mot Skills* 77 (3 Pt 1): 767–770, 1993.

Pike, R.B. *Nutrition: An Integrated Approach.* New York: Macmillan, 1984.

Quigley, M.E., and S.S.C. Yen. "The role of endogenous opiates on LH secretion during the menstrual cycle." *J Clin Endocrinol Metab* 51 (1): 179–181, 1980.

Rakatansky, H. "Chocolate: Pleasure or pain?" *Am J Psychiatry* 146 (8): 1089, 1989.

Rappoport, L., et al. "Gender and age differences in food cognition." *Appetite* 20 (1): 33–52, 1993.

Reid, L.D., and G.A. Hunter. "Morphine and naloxone modulate intake of ethanol." *Alcohol* 1 (1): 33–37, 1984.

Reid, L.D., et al. "Tests of opioid deficiency hypotheses of alcoholism." *Alcohol* 8: 247–257, 1991.

Ripsin, C.M., et al. "Oat products and lipid lowering: A meta-analysis." *JAMA* 267 (24): 3317–3325, 1992.

Sears, Barry. *The Zone.* New York: ReganBooks, 1995.

Shide, D.J., et al. "Opioid mediation of odor preferences induced by sugar and fat in 6-day-old rats." *Physiol Behav* 50 (5): 961–966, 1991.

Simopoulos, A., and J. Robinon. *The Omega Plan.* New York: HarperCollins, 1998.

Snyder, S. "The opiate receptor and morphine-like peptides in the brain." *Am J Psychiatry* 135(6): 645–652, 1978.

Somer, E. *Food & Mood.* New York: Holt, 1995.

Van der Kolk, B.A., M.S. Greenberg, S.P. Orr, and R.K. Pitman. "Endogenous opioids, stress induced analgesia, and posttraumatic stress disorder." *Psycho Pharmacol Bull* 25(3): 417–421, 1989.

Van der Kolk, B.A. *The Body Keeps Score: Memory and the Evolving Psychobiology of Posttraumatic Stress.* Boston: Massachusetts General Hospital, 1993.

Van Ree, J. "Endorphins and experimental addiction." *Alcohol* 13(1): 25, 1996.

Vanderschuren, L.J., et al. "Mu- and kappa-opioid receptor-mediated opioid effects on social play in juvenile rats." *Eur J Pharmacol* 276(3): 257–266, 1995.

Vliet, E. *Screaming to Be Heard.* New York: M. Evans, 1995.

Williams, R.J. "Alcoholism as a nutritional problem." *J Clin Nutr* 53: 32–36, 1952.

Willner, P., et al. " 'Depression' increases 'craving' for sweet rewards in animal and human models of depression and craving." *Psychopharmacology* (Berlin) 136(3): 272–283, 1998.

Wurtman, J.J., H.R. Lieberman, and B. Chew. "Changes in mood after carbohydrate consumption among obese individuals." *Am J Clin Nutr* 44: 772–778, 1986.

Wurtman, R.J., and J.J. Wurtman. "Brain serotonin, carbohydrate-craving, obesity, and depression." *Obes Res 3* (Suppl. 4): 477S–480S, 1995.

Wurtman, R.J. "Ways that foods can affect the brain." *Nutr Rev* (Supp.): 2–5, 1986.

Zorrilla, E.P., R.J. De Rubeis, and E. Redei. "High self-esteem, hardiness and affective stability are associated with higher basal pituitary-adrenal hormone levels." *Psychoneuroendocrinology* 20(6): 591–601, 1995.

Resources

Twelve-Step Programs

Addiction can take many forms. Alcoholics Anonymous is an excellent resource to guide you. Most communities have a central office of Alcoholics Anonymous. They can refer you to AA or other types of meetings more suited to your needs. They will know about:

CA (Cocaine Anonymous)
OA (Overeaters Anonymous)
Al-Anon (for families of alcoholics)
DA (Debtors Anonymous)
NA (Narcotics Anonymous)
ACOA (Adult Children of Alcoholics)
CODA (Codependents Anonymous)
SLAA (Sex and Love Addicts Anonymous)

Call local information to get your central office number, or call the national AA office at 212-870-3400.

George's Shake

George's Shake is a premade powder that provides a unique combination of protein, complex carbohydrates, vitamins, and minerals. It has no sugar, tastes wonderful, and can be an excellent support for your program. Order it from Radiant Recovery, (888) 579-3970.

Newsletter

We offer a free online newsletter through the Web site at www.radiant recovery.com.

Web Pages

Visit us at www.radiantrecovery.com. We are delighted to have your feedback and comments. Every email is answered personally. The Web page posts our scheduled appearances and lists seminars, talks, and other opportunities to meet with us. The Web page can also connect you with a number of listservs that gather people interested in special topics. Here is a partial list.

pnp12step	For those wishing to integrate twelve-step with PNP
pnpathletes	For sugar-sensitive athletes
pnpaussies	For those doing the program in Australia
pnpbigones	For people more than 100 pounds overweight
pnpbingecontrol	For sugar-sensitive bingers
pnpbrits	For those doing the program in the UK
pnpbulimia	For sugar-sensitive bulimics
pnpcollege	For sugar-sensitive college students
pnpcompassion	For those dealing with life-threatening issues
pnpdepression	For sugar-sensitive people who are depressed
pnpdiabetes	For sugar-sensitive diabetics
pnpelders	For older sugar-sensitive participants
pnpguys	For guys who are sugar sensitive
pnpjournal	For those wanting to learn how to use the food journal

pnpkiwis	For those doing the program in New Zealand
pnpoddhours	For those working irregular schedules
pnppanic	For sugar-sensitive people who are dealing with panic and anxiety
pnpparents	For parents of sugar-sensitive children
pnppets	For sugar-sensitive people with pets
pnppms	For the special needs of sugar-sensitive women
pnppregnancy	For pregnant and breast-feeding women
pnprecipes	For those wanting to share recipes
pnprecovery	For those seeking recovery from alcohol, drug, or other addiction
pnpteens	For sugar-sensitive teens
pnpvegetarians	For sugar-sensitive vegetarians
sarpbookstudy	For those interested in discussing *The Sugar Addict's Total Recovery Program* in depth

Private Consultation

Private consultations can be scheduled by emailing radiantkd@mind spring.com or calling 1(888)579-3970.

Acknowledgments

This book came from the questions and demands of sugar-sensitive people all over the world. Your needs pushed me to go further with the story of sugar sensitivity and tackle the sugar-addiction demon. Thank you for your energy, courage, and commitment. Your voices have made the book come alive with its connection to real-life stories. Thanks to all of you who cook so well and were willing to share your special recipes.

Special thanks to Margot Silk Forest for helping my vision get tucked into useful concrete specifics. I would never have done this without your help.

Thanks to Ned Leavitt for your diligence and commitment in finding a home for this wonderful story. I am deeply indebted to my editor at Ballantine, Leslie Meredith, who had the commitment to push my vision way beyond my dreams. You called the recovery voice, helped me to craft the language to give it power, and made the story come alive.

Index

adverse consequences, continued
  use despite, 17
alcohol, 44, 104, 168–69, 179
  detox, 168–69
alcoholism, 6, 7, 9, 25, 30, 31, 127,
  157, 168–69
  and beta-endorphin, 26–28, 33
  and sugar, 8, 10, 26–27, 30, 32,
    33, 165, 168–69
allergies, food, 186–87
Almonds, and Cumin, Fried Brown
  Rice with Onions, 247
ambivalence, 46, 181–82
American Psychiatric Association, 15
amino acids, 23–24, 74, 89, 92–93
anger, 4, 6, 14, 32, 135
anorexia, 72
antidepressant drugs, 23, 35, 93–95,
  210
apples, 60, 80, 85, 158
  Kathleen's Apple Carrots, 244
  Oatmeal Apple Pancakes, 217

arthritis, 97, 140
artificial sweeteners, 105, 163–64
Asian Salad, 227
Asparagus, Stir-Fried Lemon,
  242–43
aspartame, 163–64
Atkins, Robert, 36
Atkins plan, 36–37, 38

Baked Chicken and Lentils, 237
bananas, 85, 149, 190
Basic Vinaigrette, 247–48
beans, 21, 102, 134, 211
  Corn and Bean Hash, 238
  Larry's Famous Green Beans,
    243–44
beef, 74, 75, 83
  Beef Chili, 229–30
  Beef Stew, 232–33
  fast food, 199, 200
  Jeanie's Meatloaf, 234–35
  Kathleen's Meatloaf, 233–34

best way to use recovery program,
51–54
beta-endorphin, 9, 39, 41, 56, 92,
120, 151, 161, 163, 202
increasing, 41, 42, 43, 45, 56, 173,
174–75, 191–95
low, 19, 24–28, 29, 31–40, 63, 72,
191
spike triggers, 191
withdrawal, 25–28, 29, 30, 191
birthdays, 204–6
blender, 122
blood sugar volatility, 19–22, 33, 34,
40, 42, 45, 72, 87, 132, 135,
161, 207
stabilizing, 50, 74, 133, 135, 213
body language, listening to, 66–69
brain chemistry, 8, 9, 10, 14, 18,
22–40, 45, 92–97, 158, 182,
186
beta-endorphin, 19, 24–28, 29,
31–40, 41, 63, 72, 151, 163,
174–75
and dieting, 36–40
serotonin, 19, 22–24, 31–40, 73,
92–95
sex differences in, 31–33
bread, 7, 20, 34, 38, 60, 75, 132, 184,
201
Spelt and Flaxseed, 239
types of, 136
whole grain, 80, 131, 133, 134,
136, 172, 185, 213
breakfast, 19, 113–14
fast food choices, 58
importance of, 56
protein in, 42, 55–61, 71, 111,
189
recipes and suggestions, 57–58,
143, 217–21
shopping list, 59–61
skipping, 14, 34, 50, 56
breastfeeding, 80

brown foods, shifting to, 42–43,
131–49, 185–86
brown rice, 96, 134, 135, 139, 148
Brown Rice with Onions, Almonds,
and Cumin, Fried, 247
Burgers, Turkey, 226–27

Cabbage, Scalloped, 244
caffeine, 44, 55, 164
cake, 132, 135, 147, 160
birthday, 204–6
Carrot Cake, 249–50
Pumpkin Cake with Cashew
Butter Frosting, 251
Pumpkin Tofu Cheesecake,
250
car, eating in the, 208–10
carbohydrates, 43
complex, 7, 72, 78, 80, 105, 162,
172, 185, 212, 213
and dieting, 36–40
sensitivity, 19–22, 33–36
carrots, 84, 123, 124
Carrot Cake, 249–50
Kathleen's Apple Carrots, 244
Cashew Butter Frosting, Pumpkin
Cake with, 251
Casserole, Chili Layered, 229
cereal, 20, 75, 85, 132
options, 136–39
see also oatmeal
C57 mice research, 26–28
cheating, 5
cheese, 60, 80, 82, 83, 104, 124,
128
Feta Frittata, 225–26
Feta-Walnut Spread for Veggies
or Sandwiches, 224–25
Pumpkin Tofu Cheesecake, 250
Ricotta Fruit "Pudding," 252
Yogurt Ricotta Delight, 218
Cheesecake, Pumpkin Tofu, 250
chicken, 74, 75, 83, 102

Baked Chicken and Lentils, 237–38
Chicken Meatloaf, 235
Chicken Roasted with Garlic, 231–32
fast food, 199, 200
Kathleen's Roast Chicken with Vegetables, 232
Roast Sticky Chicken, 230–31
chili, 202
Beef Chili, 229–30
Chili Layered Casserole, 229
Chinese food, 163, 200–201
chocolate, 14, 33, 203
Christmas, without sugars, 176–78, 203
cigarette smoking, 11, 44
Cinnamon–Cottage Cheese Pancakes, 217–18
coffee, 29, 44, 55, 80, 120
colored markers, use of, 51–52
comfort, creating other kinds of, 190–95
comfort foods, 105–6, 133
new, 146–49
compassion, 112
contingency plans, making, 196–97
cooking, 47, 103–4, 118
methods, 121–22
corn, 84, 124, 146
Corn and Bean Hash, 238
corn syrup, 160
cottage cheese, 60, 75, 76, 82, 83, 85, 102
Cottage Cheese–Cinnamon Pancakes, 217–18
covert sugars, 151, 152, 153, 160–63
crankiness, what to do about, 185–87
crashing, 111–14, 127–28
criteria for addiction, 15–18

Crock-Pot, 121
Crustless Quiche, 221–30

dairy products, 75, 83
depression, 6, 9, 14, 22–23, 35, 47, 70, 210
and brain chemistry, 22–23, 32, 92–95
dessert:
recipes, 149, 248–52
saying no to, 179–80
detox, sugar, 150–75, 186, 190, 212
attentiveness to plan, 164–67
final preparations, 169–71
life after, 174–75
and spotting sugars, 159–64
what to eat, 171–74
diabetes, 20–21, 96, 212–13
diets, 7, 36–40
Atkins plan, 36–37, 38
Hellers' plan, 38–39
ineffective in sugar addicts, 36–40
Protein Power, 37–38
Zone, 37, 38
dinner recipes and suggestions, 143–45, 230–38
dopamine, 163–64
downtimes, planning for, 126–30
dreams, 94, 100, 140
dressings, 129, 247–48
Basic Vinaigrette, 247–48
Fried Eggplant with Yogurt-Garlic Dressing, 245
Simple Salad Dressing, 248
drug addiction, 6, 7, 9, 25, 30

Eades, Michael and Mary Dan, 37
Easy Egg and Oat One-Pan Breakfast, 219
eating alone, 103
eat-on-the-run type, 117

Eggplant with Yogurt-Garlic
    Dressing, Fried, 245
eggs, 55, 58, 59, 60, 75, 78, 80, 82,
    83, 85, 102, 125
    Crustless Quiche, 221–22
    Easy Egg and Oat One-Pan
        Breakfast, 219
    Feta Frittata, 225–26
    Italian Frittata, 236
    Potato-Crusted Quiche, With or
        Without Meat, 222–23
emergency foods, 82
exercise, 102, 118–19, 165, 166–67,
    192, 193, 194

family, 202
    help from, 183–84
    saying no to, 178–81
    talking to, 154–55
fast foods, 58, 129–30, 199–200
fatigue, 6, 188
fats, 20, 22, 36–37, 90–91
    in diet, 90–91
fear, 109
Feta Frittata, 225–26
Feta-Walnut Spread for Veggies or
    Sandwiches, 224–25
fiber, 20, 22, 41, 96, 132, 133, 158
finances, 102–3
fish, 74, 75, 76, 83, 102
    Salmon Patties, 237
5HTP, 104
flags, use of, 52–53
Flaxseed and Spelt Bread, 239
food journal, see journal, food
foreign foods, 200–202
Foster-Powell, Kaye, 21–22
Fried Brown Rice with Onions,
    Almonds, and Cumin, 247
Fried Eggplant with Yogurt-Garlic
    Dressing, 245
friends, 205
    help from, 183–84

saying no to, 178–81
talking to, 154–55
Frittata, Feta, 225–26
Frittata, Italian, 236
frozen food, 122
fruits, 60, 85, 137, 158, 209
    Ricotta Fruit "Pudding," 252
functional/factual type, 116
fuzzy food syndrome, 86

garlic:
    Chicken Roasted with Garlic,
        231–32
    Fried Eggplant with Yogurt-Garlic
        Dressing, 245
George's Shake, 57, 58, 105, 129,
    208, 220–21, 264
Gianoulakis, Dr. Christine, 26
glucose, 166, 212
glycemic index (GI), 20–22, 87,
    96–97
graceful refusal, art of, 178–81
granola, 137
Great Potato Soup, 240
Green Beans, Larry's Famous,
    243–44
grocery shopping, 59–61, 81–86
    for three meals a day with
        protein, 81–86

hangover, sugar, 5, 16
Hash, Corn and Bean, 238
headaches, 5, 40, 93, 94, 151
Heller, Richard and Rachel,
    38–39
Hellers' plan, 38–39
herbs, 89, 104
heroin, 9, 25
holidays, 176–78, 202–4
honey, 160
hopelessness, 13, 23, 30, 32
hyperactivity, 27
hypoglycemia, 19

ice cream, 78, 160
"I don't want to change" type, 116
"I eat if you fix it" type, 117–18
impulse control, lack of, 6, 7, 14,
    22–24, 31, 32, 34, 79
Indian food, 201
indoor grills, 121
insulin, 19–20, 24, 41, 87, 92, 93, 96,
    118, 161, 212
    and dieting, 36–40
Internet, 184–85
Italian food, 201–2
Italian Frittata, 236

Japanese food, 201
Jeanie's Meatloaf, 234–35
Jenkins, David, 20–21
journal, food, 42, 47, 61–69, 108,
    110–14, 134, 150, 158, 159,
    161, 164, 185, 208

Kathleen's Apple Carrots, 244
Kathleen's Meatloaf, 233–34
Kathleen's Roast Chicken with
    Vegetables, 232
kitchen, cleaning your, 153–54

labels, food, 161–63
lamb, 75
Larry's Famous Green Beans,
    243–44
Lemon Asparagus, Stir-Fried,
    242–43
Lemon Potatoes, Roasted, 241
lentils, 21, 75, 102, 134
    Baked Chicken and Lentils,
    237–38
lettuce, 84
listening, 114
    to your body, 66–69
love, 152
lunch recipes, 221–30
lying, 4, 5

maltodextrin, 162
maple syrup, 160
margins, writing in, 53
mastery, 115
meals:
    definition of, 77–78
    examples of, 77
    overdue, 79
    sweets with, 78
    three a day, with protein, 42, 51,
    71–86, 95, 99, 108, 189
    see also breakfast; dinner; lunch
meat, see beef; chicken; lamb;
    sausage; turkey
meatloaf, 123–24
    Chicken, 235
    Jeanie's, 234–35
    Kathleen's, 233–34
    Soy, 235–36
meditation, 192
men, 45, 46
    brain chemicals in, 31–33
menopause, 33, 97
menstrual cycle, 32–33
Mexican food, 202
Microwave Nut Butter Oatmeal,
    219
milk, 83, 98, 158
minerals, 88
    zinc, 88, 165, 166
molasses, 160
mood swings, 6, 7–8, 14, 20, 35, 45,
    68, 69, 101
morphine, 27
Muffins, Oatmeal, 220
munchies, 128

new life, creating, 43, 50, 176–95
newsletter, 264
no, saying, 178–82
notebook, setting up a, 53–54
Nut Butter Oatmeal, Microwave, 219
nuts, 128, 129

OA (Overeaters Anonymous), 101–2
oatmeal, 21, 82, 85, 96, 134, 137–39
    benefits of, 137–39
    Easy Egg and Oat One-Plan
        Breakfast, 219
    Microwave Nut Butter Oatmeal,
        219
    Oatmeal Apple Pancakes, 217
    Oatmeal Muffins, 220
one-pot meals, 116, 121, 145, 185–86
Onions, Almonds, and Cumin, Fried
    Brown Rice with, 247
online support, 184–85
opioids, 9–10
optimism, 115
oranges, 85
orgasm, 93
oven, 122
Oven-Fried Sweet Potatoes, 141–42,
    245–46
overt sugars, 151, 153, 159–60
ovulation, 32, 33

pain tolerance, low, 31, 34
pancakes:
    Cottage Cheese–Cinnamon,
        217–18
    Oatmeal Apple, 217
pasta, 7, 34, 132, 158, 198, 201
    alternatives, 139–40
Patties, Salmon, 237
peaches, 85
peanut butter, 60, 75, 80, 102
    Squash Pie with Peanut Butter
        Glaze, 248–49
peas, 84, 124, 146
perfection, 188
pets, 192, 193
phenylalanine, 163–64
Pie with Peanut Butter Glaze,
    Squash, 248–49
pizza, 147
plane trips, 208

planning your food, 115–18
PMS, 6, 32, 33
Post-it notes, use of, 52
potato, 20, 21, 24, 60, 82, 84, 85,
    86–88, 92–101, 124, 134,
    140–42, 184, 209, 213
    and brain chemistry, 24, 87,
        92–97
    choice and preparation of,
        97–99, 141–42
    Great Potato Soup, 240
    how it works, 92–97
    nightly, 42, 50, 86–88, 92–101,
        108, 128
    Oven-Fried Sweet Potatoes,
        141–42, 245–46
    Potato-Crusted Quiche, With or
        Without Meat, 222–23
    Roasted Lemon Potatoes, 241
    Roast Potatoes, 241
    size of, 93–94, 98
    skin, 87, 134
    Spicy Oven-Fried Potatoes, 242
    Sweet Potato Pie, 247
    Sweet Potato Puff, 246
    timing of, 99–101
    types of, 86–88
Potatoes Not Prozac (DesMaisons),
    10–11, 24, 43, 96, 143, 186
pregnancy, 80, 211–12
protein, 7, 20, 36, 41, 91–92, 105,
    158, 185, 198, 212
    amounts of, 91–92
    in breakfast, 42, 55–61, 71, 111,
        189
    costs of, 102–3
    and dieting, 36–40
    regular, 41, 73–77
    snacks, 71–72
    three meals a day with, 42, 51,
        71–86, 95, 99, 108, 189
    and tryptophan, 23–24, 92–93
Protein Power diet, 37–38

protein shakes, 57, 58, 76, 77, 105, 129, 208, 220–21
Prozac, 23
pumpkin:
Pumpkin Cake with Cashew Butter Frosting, 251
Pumpkin Tofu Cheesecake, 250

quiche:
Crustless, 221–22
Potato-Crusted Quiche, With or Without Meat, 222–23

radiance, reaching, 43, 50, 176–95
recipes, 148, 216–52
bread, 239
breakfast, 142–43, 217–21
desserts, 149, 248–52
dinner, 143–45, 230–38
lunch, 221–30
salad dressings, 247–48
soup and side dishes, 240–47
trying new, 125–26
see also specific recipes
recommended daily allowance (RDA), 91
red wine, 104
reframing, 151, 178
refusal, art of, 178–81
relapse, 110–14, 175, 187–91
getting back to the plan, 189–90
warning signs, 188
resources, 263–65
responsibilities, sugar interference with, 16
restaurants, 163, 184, 197–202
asking for what you want in, 198–99
fast food, 58, 129–30, 199–200
rice, 20, 132
Fried Brown Rice with Onions, Almonds, and Cumin, 247
rice cakes, 85, 96

rice cooker, 121
Ricotta Delight, Yogurt, 218
Ricotta Fruit "Pudding," 252
Roasted Lemon Potatoes, 241
Roast Potatoes, 241
Roast Sticky Chicken, 230–31
routine, creating a, 107–30

sadness, 156–57
St. John's wort, 104
salad, 198, 199
Asian Salad, 227
dressings, 129, 247–48
fast food, 199, 200
Simple Tofu Salad, 228–29
T 'n' T Salad, 228
type, 117
salmon, 75, 76
Salmon Patties, 237
Feta-Walnut Spread for, 224–25
sausage, 55
Potato-Crusted Quiche, With or Without Meat, 222–23
Scalloped Cabbage, 244
Sears, Barry, 37
seasonal affective disorder (SAD), 23, 94
second thoughts, 156–57
self-esteem, 25, 45
low, 8, 9, 32, 33
and opioids, 9–10
serotonin, 41, 76, 92, 114, 120, 166
increasing, 41, 42, 45, 92–95, 140
low, 19, 22–24, 31–40, 73, 87
sex, 192
sex differences in brain chemicals, 31–33
sex drive, lack of, 35
Shake, George's, 57, 58, 105, 129, 208, 220–21, 264
side dishes, 240–47
Simple Salad Dressing, 248
Simple Tofu Salad, 228–29

simplicity, importance of, 48–51
sleep, 94, 100, 140
slipping, 110–14, 127–28, 175,
    187–88
slowing down, 54
snacks, 79–80, 102
    protein, 71–72
social activity, 80
    decrease in, 17
    without sugars, 176–81
soda, 16, 80, 120, 160, 164
solution to sugar addiction, 41–54
soup, 85
    Great Potato Soup, 240
soy, 21, 75
    Soy Meatloaf, 235–36
    see also tofu
special situations, 196–215
    antidepressants, 210
    diabetes, 212–13
    holidays and birthdays, 202–6
    pregnancy, 211–12
    restaurants, 197–202
    traveling, 206–11
    vegetarians, 210–11
Spelt and Flaxseed Bread, 239
spelt flour, 136
Spicy Oven-Fried Potatoes, 242
spotting sugars, 159–64
Spread, Feta-Walnut, 224–25
Squash Pie with Peanut Butter
    Glaze, 248–49
stability, 70–89, 150, 158
    creating a routine, 107–30
    staying out of trouble, 182–83
stealing, 5
Step 1, 42, 55–61
Step 2, 42, 61–69
Step 3, 42, 51, 71–86
Step 4, 42, 50, 86–89, 91–101
Step 5, 42–43, 131–49
Step 6, 43, 150–75
Step 7, 43, 50, 176–95

Stew, Beef, 232–33
Stir-Fried Lemon Asparagus, 242–43
style, detox, 169–70
sugar, taking out the, 43, 150–75
sugar addiction, definition of, 3–5,
    15–18
Sugar Busters! program, 40
sugar feelings, 47–48
    managing intensity of, 68–69
sugar sensitivity, 10, 11, 14, 18, 40,
    186–87
    and brain chemicals, 22–40, 41
    and carbohydrates, 19–22,
        33–36
    components of, 18–36
    definition of, 10, 11
support, getting, 183–85
sushi, 201
Sweet Potatoes, Oven-Fried, 141–42,
    245–46
Sweet Potato Pie, 247
Sweet Potato Puff, 246

tea, 80, 120
tempeh, 211
Thai food, 201
three meals a day with protein, 42,
    51, 71–86, 95, 99, 108, 189
time, detox, 169, 171
T 'n' T Salad, 228
toaster oven, 121
tofu, 75, 83, 102, 210–11
    Feta Frittata, 225–26
    Pumpkin Tofu Cheesecake, 250
    Simple Tofu Salad, 228–29
    Tofu Scramble, 223–24
tolerance, increase in, 17
tomato, 84
traveling, 206–11
Triscuits, 60, 80, 82, 96, 127, 128,
    129, 146–47, 213
trouble, staying out of, 182–83
Trout, David, 21

tryptophan, 23–24, 36, 76, 87,
92–93, 114, 166
tuna, 75, 82, 83, 207
T 'n' T Salad, 228
turkey, 75, 76, 83, 102
Turkey Burgers, 226–27
twelve-step programs, 7, 46, 155,
263
tyrosine, 104

unsuccessful attempts to cut down
on sugar, 16

Valentine's Day, 203
vegetables, 59, 75, 82, 83–84,
122–25, 146, 164–65, 172,
185–86, 198, 199, 209,
210–11
Feta-Walnut Spread for,
224–25
Kathleen's Roast Chicken with
Vegetables, 232
side dishes, 241–47
see also salad; specific vegetables and
recipes
vegetarians, 75, 210–11
Vinaigrette, Basic, 247–48
vitamins, 42, 88–89, 108, 114,
165–66
B complex, 88, 165, 166
C, 88, 165–66

Walnut-Feta Spread for Veggies or
Sandwiches, 224–25
water, drinking, 119–20, 165,
166–67, 209
Web sites, 48, 184, 264–65
weight gain, 6, 7, 8, 34, 101–2
and dieting, 36–40
white flour foods, 5, 22, 30, 44, 68,
132, 151, 172, 191
shifting to brown foods, 42–43,
131–49, 185–86
whole grains, 41, 80, 133, 172, 185,
213
shifting to, 42–43, 131–49, 185–86
wine, red, 104
withdrawal, 15, 16, 25, 30, 40
beta-endorphin, 25–28, 29, 30, 191
symptoms, 17
use to prevent, 17–18
women, 45, 46
brain chemistry in, 32–33

yoga, 192
yogurt, 83, 102
Fried Eggplant with Yogurt-Garlic
Dressing, 245
Yogurt Ricotta Delight, 218

zinc, 88, 165, 166
Zoloft, 23
Zone plan, 37, 38

About the Author

KATHLEEN DESMAISONS, PH.D., revolutionized the field of chemical dependency treatment with her pioneering work in addictive nutrition. In her best-selling book, *Potatoes Not Prozac,* she coined the term "sugar sensitivity" to describe a common biochemical tendency toward addiction, depression, and obesity. Her dietary recommendations have offered simple solutions with profound results for people who have followed uncountable "diets" without long-lasting success.

A graduate of the Union Institute, Dr. DesMaisons created her field of study, earning the first degree ever awarded in addictive nutrition. She currently lives in Albuquerque, New Mexico, where she serves as President/CEO of Radiant Recovery, maintains a private consulting practice, and nurtures a thriving online community. Thousands of her readers regularly contribute to the exceptionally welcoming Web site (www.radiant recovery.com), together creating a safe and supportive circle for sugar addicts seeking recovery. Dr. DesMaisons can be reached by email at kathleen@radiantrecovery.com.